# THE BIBLE CURE

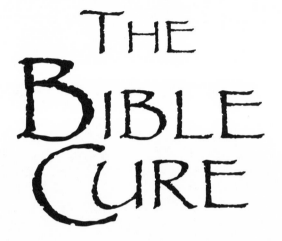

# REGINALD CHERRY, M.D.

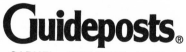

CARMEL • NEW YORK 10512

www.guideposts.org

Unless otherwise noted, all Scripture quotations are from the King James Version of the Bible.

Scripture quotations marked AMP are from the Amplified Bible. Old Testament copyright © 1965, 1987 by the Zondervan Corporation. The Amplified New Testament copyright © 1954, 1958, 1987 by the Lockman Foundation. Used by permission.

Scripture quotations marked NIV are from the Holy Bible, New International Version. Copyright © 1973, 1978, 1984, International Bible Society. Used by permission.

Scripture quotations marked NLT are from the Holy Bible, New Living Translation, copyright © 1996. Used by permission of Tyndale House Publishers, Inc., Wheaton, IL 60189. All rights reserved.

Scripture quotations marked NAS are from the New American Standard Bible. Copyright © 1960, 1962, 1963, 1968, 1971, 1972, 1973, 1975, 1977 by the Lockman Foundation. Used by permission.

Scripture quotations marked RSV are from the Revised Standard Version of the Bible. Copyright © 1946, 1952, 1971 by the Division of Christian Education of the National Council of the Churches of Christ in the USA. Used by permission.

Copyright © 1998 by Reginald Cherry
All rights reserved.

**Library of Congress Cataloging-in-Publication Data**
Cherry, Reginald B.
    The Bible cure / Reginald B. Cherry.
       p.  cm.
    ISBN: 0–88419–535–X (alk. paper)
    1. Health. 2. Medicine in the Bible. 3. Nutrition. 4. Medicine,
Popular.  I. Title.
RA776.5.C4715 1998                         98–15698
613—dc21                                 CIP

*Printed in the United States of America*

This book is dedicated
to all of our patients who have
received their healing through the Bible cure
and to all of our future patients and readers who
*will* receive their healing through
*The Bible Cure*.

# Contents

# Foreword

WITHIN THE ANCIENT Greek, Aramaic, and Hebrew texts of the sacred Judeo-Christian Scriptures mysteriously lies *the Bible Cure*. Within the Bible's holy writ are all the principles needed by each of us to find healing for body, soul, and spirit. Like rough, uncut gems hidden within the ore of a deep mine, these jewels of the Bible cure can be mined, revealed, refined, and brilliantly displayed in our lives to the glory of the God who fearfully and wonderfully created us.

Together, you and I will walk through *The Bible Cure* and uncover the secrets of God's pathway of healing for you. God has revealed the principles of the Bible cure to me as a Christian medical doctor. I have witnessed how the Bible cure has changed my life as a practicing physician and the lives of my patients as they have applied Bible cure truths to their lives. Many of these patients had been diagnosed with incurable diseases before they ever came to me.

I have seen the Bible cure work for patients afflicted with:

- Cancer
- Heart disease
- High blood pressure
- Diabetes
- Fatigue
- Genetic defects
- Skin diseases
- Even the annoyances of allergies

I have seen God heal almost every major disease through His Bible cure in this practice of medicine, including some very rare illnesses.

The principles of *The Bible Cure* include deciphering the ancient Hebrew dietary laws; understanding how Jesus anointed natural substances to heal; and how we can pray specifically for healing and overcoming the mountain of our illness.

Are you ready to discover your Bible cure? Join me for this exciting journey along your pathway of healing.

—*REGINALD B. CHERRY, M.D.*

# 1

# Truths That Amazed
# This Scientist and Physician

WOVEN INTO ANCIENT Hebrew, Aramaic, and Greek manuscripts are clues to health and healing only recently validated by scientific and medical research. As a young, premed student at Baylor University, and later in medical school at the University of Texas at San Antonio, I became curious about the ancient texts now called the Bible and their relationship to modern-day medicine.

I am a medical doctor educated and trained at one of the University of Texas Medical Schools and licensed to practice medicine in the state of Texas. I am equipped to be a scientist and a physician specializing in the field of preventive medicine.

As I see patients daily, I am constantly amazed by the findings of medical science and the power of faith and prayer working together to reveal the Bible cure for patients.

Yes, I said, *Bible cure*. Before I was a Christian, I was a science major in premed at Baylor University. Even then, I was astonished by the ways dietary and nutritional laws given in the ancient biblical texts revealed truths that scientists were only beginning to uncover in this century.

## THE MYSTERY OF CARBOHYDRATES AND FATS

LET ME GIVE you an example of how the Bible cure and present-day science reveal pathways of healing and health for us right now. One big issue that has baffled scientists and physicians for years is the role that carbohydrates and fats play in our diet and health.

For many years, many experts in the field of medicine thought that a high-carbohydrate diet was the ideal diet. Others believed a vegetarian diet to be the ideal diet. In more recent studies, scientists have found there are some detrimental aspects to an all-vegetarian diet. Likewise, scientists used to think that the lower the fat intake, the healthier we would be. However, current research has uncovered the fact that eliminating all fat is not the healthiest way to eat. In fact, we need certain fats in our diet.

The Bible cure addressed the issues of how carbohydrates and fats affect our health thousands of years before the birth of Christ. In the Massoretic texts of the Torah, we can decipher two diets. The Hebrew text for Genesis 1:29 describes the first diet: על־פני כל־הארץ ואת־כל־העץ אשר־בו פרי־עץ זרע זרע לכם ויאמר אלהים הנה נתתי לכם את־כל־עשׂב זרע זרע אשר (Gen. 1:29). The Amplified Bible translates this command from God to read, "And God said, See, I have given you every plant yielding seed that is on the face of all the land, and every tree with seed in its fruit; you shall have them for food."

This first diet focuses on:

- Every herb-bearing seed (את־כל־עשׂב זרע זרע). Eating plants and seeds—the whole grain and not the bleached germ of the seed—is central to the Bible cure's code for ingesting healthy food. This included grains and some legumes that help to lower harmful cholesterol levels and protect against high blood pressure. Such a diet is low in sodium and rich in potassium.

- Fruit of a seed-yielding tree (פרי־עץ זרע זרע). As we shall see later in this book, fruits are loaded with soluble fiber, the benefit of which is to lower cholesterol levels. Also, the soluble fiber in fruits as well as in certain vegetables speeds up the elimination of harmful substances from our bodies that increase our risk of cancer.

- " . . . shall be for meat [food]" (יהיה לאכלה). The word for *meat* (אכל) is the basic Hebrew noun for *food*—not meat. This dietary instruction from God is a general instruction that the first diet of food consists of fruit, seeds, plants, or herbs; it does not refer to substituting meat for vegetables.

Later in Genesis we observe how God adds meat protein to our diets. In the second diet prescribed in the Torah, God adds another source of protein to our diets: עשב נתתי לכם את־כל כל־רמש אשר הוא־חי לכם יהיה לאכלה כירק (Gen. 9:3). God allows meat to be consumed as protein by commanding, "Every moving thing that lives shall be food for you; and as I give you the green vegetables and plants, I give you everything" (Gen. 9:3, AMP). This isn't a new diet but simply an extension of His command in Genesis 1:29. First, we are given plant food (עשב), seeds (זרע), and fruit of a tree (פרי־עץ) to eat. To that, in Genesis 9:3 God adds every moving thing that lives (כל־רמש אשר הוא־חי). God restricts certain foods, which we will later see in Leviticus and Deuteronomy.

It is intriguing to study diets around the world today from Mexico, the Far East, and the Near East, and to discover that when their diets closely parallel the Bible cure's edicts for food, they live healthier and longer lives on average than Americans who have added so many processed foods and fat to our diets.

One interesting study focused on the Bantu tribe in Africa. One Bantu group ate a purely vegetarian diet, incorporating only part of the Bible cure from Genesis 1:29. This group, with plants as an essential, predominant part of their diet, were receiving the carbohydrates that they needed but lacked necessary protein.

3

A second group from the tribe lived near a large lake and ate large amounts of fish—but no other meat. The study discovered that the vegetarians had higher blood levels of the bad low-density lipoproteins (LDL cholesterol), while the fish eaters had an average 40 percent lower level of the LDL cholesterol found in plants. The fish eaters who were following the Bible cure in Genesis 9:3 were healthy, living longer, and had a lower incidence of heart disease. Why? They had higher levels of a beneficial form of cholesterol called *high-density lipoproteins (HDL)*, which, at appropriate levels, is actually good for us. Therefore, this study clearly indicates that eating meat such as fish and chicken can actually enhance our health and lower our risk for some forms of diseases.

## *LDL and HDL in Heart Disease*

℞ The villain in heart disease is LDL, the "bad" form of cholesterol. (HDL is the "good" or protective component.) LDL is deposited into the wall of the arteries as it circulates in the bloodstream, where it stimulates chemical changes that lead to the formation of atherosclerotic plaques. This harmful process is aggravated by free radicals in the area—end products of oxygen metabolism in the body. (Free radicals are analogous to the exhaust of a car. They have negative effects, including this effect on LDL in the arterial wall.)[1]

Let me give you another example of how the Bible cure interfaces with modern-day science as research gleans new information about living and eating healthy. In Leviticus 3:17, there is a general prohibition against eating fat. But the Bible cure becomes very specific in Leviticus 7:23–24: ואכל לא תאכלהו
כל־חלב שור וכשב ועז לא תאכלו וחלב נבלה וחלב טרפה יעשה לכל־מלאכה
דבר אל־בני ישראל לאמר

The Amplified translation of this ancient Semitic text reads, "Say to the Israelites, You shall eat no kind of fat, of ox, or sheep, or goat. The fat of the beast that dies of itself, and the fat of one that is torn with beasts, may be put to any other use, but under no circumstances are you to eat of it."

So we see God's prohibition against fat. But why is it that throughout the Bible we see so many mentions of olives and olive oil, which are extremely high in fat? Even today in Israel they use a lot of olives and olive oil. When you look carefully at the Genesis and Leviticus Scriptures, you can see that God is talking about "saturated fat"—He describes fat from animals, not from plants. The Hebrew of Leviticus is very specific about the fat it is describing. This fat—(חלב)—does not refer to the fat grams found in plants, but specifically to the fat from animal sacrifices. It's amazing to understand that the ancient texts, recorded by people who had no knowledge of modern science or medicine, are very specific and accurate about the Bible cure. God not only revealed that fat would be harmful to eat, but He also named the specific kind of fat that was most harmful, using the exact word for that fat—(חלב)—animal fat!

---

### חלב *Fat in Hebrew*

א This Hebrew word usually refers to the fat of animals or "midriff fat." The fat of sacrificial animals, specifically the fat surrounding the kidneys and intestines, was burned by the priests. (See Leviticus 3:3–4, 10, 14–16.) In some cases the fat tail of the broadtail sheep, which can weigh up to ten pounds, was offered. (See Leviticus 3:9; Exodus 29:22.)

Fat was burned in the following offerings:

1. The "burnt offering" (KJV) or holocaust. (See Leviticus 1:8, 12, where *peder,* "suet," is used.)
2. The "peace offering" (KJV) or "fellowship offering" (NIV). (See Leviticus 3:9; 7:15.)
3. The "sin offering" (Lev. 4:8–10).
4. The "trespass offering" (KJV) or "guilt offering" (NIV) (Lev. 7:3–4).

Like the blood, the fat was not to be eaten (Lev. 3:17; 7:23, 25).[2]

---

This raises an interesting question. For many years, physicians, nutritionists, and scientists have held to the general assumption that people should be on a low-fat diet, the lower the better. But when one carefully examines the Bible cure in the Hebrew and Aramaic manuscripts, one sees constant mention of high-fat foods that are not meat products such as olives and olive oil. A few examples are given below:

- "And houses full of all good things, which thou filledst not, and wells digged, which thou diggedst not, vineyards and olive trees, which thou plantedst not; when thou shalt have eaten and be full" (Deut. 6:11).

- "A land of wheat, and barley, and vines, and fig trees, and pomegranates; a land of oil olive, and honey" (Deut. 8:8).

- "Thy wife shall be as a fruitful vine by the sides of thine house: thy children like olive plants round about thy table" (Ps. 128:3).

- "His branches shall spread, and his beauty shall be as the olive tree, and his smell as Lebanon" (Hos. 14:6).

Olive oil and olives have a completely different kind of fat called *monosaturated fat,* which is different from the saturated fats in animals. What's so different about monosaturated fat? It lowers the level of bad cholesterol (LDL) and boosts the level of good cholesterol (HDL), and it enhances the body's immune system function.

Lynne Scott, R.D., director of the Diet Modification Clinic at Baylor College of Medicine in Houston, says:

> These monounsaturated oils don't seem to lower the good HDL (high-density lipoprotein) cholesterol the way polyunsaturates like corn, safflower, and sesame oil can. I highly recommend olive oil for things like salads, and milder-tasting canola oil for baking, to take the place of butter and lard. Monounsaturates may also protect LDL cholesterol from oxidation, a chemical change that can lead to clogged arteries and heart attacks.[3]

So now science has begun to say, "Wait a minute. We have gone too far with this fat restriction thing. People need fat in their diet." Today we consider the basic diet of the ancient Hebrews—the Mediterranean Diet—as the ideal diet for health. I will share this diet with you in depth in chapter three.

Monosaturated fat predominates in the Mediterranean Diet; it is found in such foods as olives, nuts, and other healthy foods such as barley. (See Genesis 43:11; Numbers 11:5; Deuteronomy 8; Proverbs 25:16.)

We will also discover why the Bible cure forbids eating such meat as pork and shellfish while allowing meat such as certain fish, poultry, and beef. I will be excited to share with you how to make the very healthy bread of Ezekiel. The Bible cure is not a manual of nutrition, but it is a guide, found in the ancient biblical text, to your pathway of healing. God did not set out to write a nutritional manual. But a person who perceptively and rightly divides the Word can dissect out a cure and pathway of healing that God has planned for His people. And every single thing we are discovering in science today parallels and bolsters what the Bible says about nutrition.

Through the New Covenant we now have the ability to overcome the damage caused to our health by poor dietary and lifestyle habits. But we cannot reverse God's health laws. For example, we know that we cannot get all the nutrients we need from the plant kingdom—iron and $B_{12}$ are just two examples. Soy is the only source of complete protein from plants, and most people around the world find it difficult to eat soy products. Therefore, to get a complete protein from the plant kingdom alone, we are forced to combine certain foods. But by simply adding a piece of fish or chicken, which are low in the saturated fats, to our diets, we can get the necessary protein instantly.

Thousands of years before we had any knowledge of LDL and HDL cholesterol, the Bible cure indicated that certain foods, including meats, could be eaten, giving specific health benefits to our bodies and lifestyles. As we unravel these ancient texts and explore modern science and medicine, we will discover how our pathway to healing will include God's ancient dietary laws, *Jehovah Rapha's* revelations and teachings about healing, and the use of today's medicines and natural substances to healing and health.

## LIFE SPAN AND THE BIBLE CURE

GERONTOLOGY IS THE medical science that studies aging. Long before we had any scientific evidence about how long we should live, the Bible cure gave specific answers and insights. Scientists have been trying to unravel the mysteries of aging for decades. In the early fifties, Leonard Hayflick, a scientist at the University of California, San Francisco, discovered a very interesting thing: All human cells are able to reproduce themselves only a certain number of times. This is estimated to be about fifty cell divisions, which Dr. Hayflick estimated would place the human life at between one hundred fifteen and one hundred twenty years.[4] Researchers still don't know what drives this cellular timetable, but the life span of humans seems to be set at approximately one hundred twenty years. Researchers can study a culture of human cells as they divide repeatedly until a maximum of fifty to sixty divisions, which equates to one hundred twenty years.

Centuries before Hayflick, the Bible cure had already revealed the life span of humans in Genesis 6:3: מאה ועשׂרים שׁנה והיו ימיו or translated, " . . . yet his days shall be an hundred and twenty years." Our pathway of healing as identified in the Bible cure has already been prescribed at one hundred twenty years. Science has uncovered an ancient truth revealed by God thousands of years ago. This is just one more example to whet your appetite for joining me in the study of the Bible cure in the coming pages.

Before we closely examine the ancient Hebrew and Greek texts that reveal the Bible cure, let me share with you how God (Jehovah God) led me from being a curious student of religion to a committed Christian who believes that God reveals His Bible cure to us through our own personal pathway of healing.

## FROM SCIENTIST AND PHYSICIAN TO CHRISTIAN DOCTOR

MY JOURNEY TOWARD uncovering the Bible cure began in medical school. I was not a Christian at that time, but I was drawn regularly to watch Billy Graham's crusades on television and to reading the Bible on occasion. My curiosity about the relationship between Scripture and medicine began to intensify years later, however.

I had read over the years various Scriptures such as David talking about how we are "fearfully and wonderfully made." I also remember reading about how the eye is the light of the soul. In medical school, during the physical examination course, I was awed when we studied the human eye. I discovered that it was, in fact, the only place in the body that arteries, veins, and even the end of a nerve (the optic nerve) could be observed directly. We further learned that by examining the eye, a doctor could detect over two hundred different diseases in the human body. These were astounding medical insights to me and I couldn't help but think of how God truly did make the human body in a "fearful and wonderful" way.

After medical school and residency, I began seeing patients who had real problems. These were not textbook cases but flesh and blood human beings who hurt, felt deeply, and from time to time died, even though I used the best medical knowledge to try to heal them.

When I finally accepted the Lord in 1979 and was born into His kingdom, I was already beginning to understand that there had to be a source of healing beyond what scientific knowledge and medicine offers to heal people. I read that God was *Jehovah Rapha* (אני יהוה רפא)—"I am the LORD that healeth thee" (Exod. 15:26). God revealed to me the existence of a pathway of healing in which God uses both the natural and the supernatural to heal. (See John 9:1–7; Mark 10:46–52.)

After I was saved I worshiped in a small church that believed in God's healing power and in praying for the sick (James 5:16). I began noticing that people were being healed supernaturally at church.

One of the first healings I observed after being saved was a lady with severe back problems. Back problems can be very challenging in the practice of medicine because physicians often don't have many effective treatments to offer that can help. We give painkillers and hope that with time the back problems will disappear. But this lady had suffered for a long time. In one church service, people gathered around her, laid hands on her, and prayed. Suddenly her back pain disappeared.

At first I thought, *This is just an emotional thing*. I believed that her back problems would soon return after the excitement of the moment ebbed away. But the next Sunday arrived and she was still healed and had no pain. The next month rolled around, and she was still free from pain. As I watched this woman who had been in so much pain come to church month after month completely healed, the reality that God heals began to be confirmed to me.

Later, we began attending Lakewood Church in Houston, Texas. In one evening service, we noticed a man walking on crutches in the back of the sanctuary. No one laid hands on this man or prayed specifically for him, but the pastor spoke by revelation knowledge that someone with back pain was being healed by God. Our pastor affirmed, "If you will accept your healing, you will be healed right now."

Suddenly this man started yelling. A commotion of noise arose all around him. I was still very young in my Christian faith, but I was open to the reality that God willed to heal people today. So I watched this man on the crutches with both spiritual anticipation and medical curiosity. He simply put his crutches under his arms, ran down the aisle, and climbed up the steps to the platform where our pastor was standing.

The entire audience was electrified. This man's family joined him and confirmed the extent of his disability, rejoicing, with tears, at how whole God had made him. They said, "Since childhood, he's never been able to walk more than a few steps without excruciating pain, much less run. He hasn't run since he was a little kid. He has been on crutches for years. Orthopedic surgeons have given up on him, telling him he would never walk without assistance again."

The man who had been crippled was now running all over the platform to demonstrate to everyone that God had really healed him. I witnessed the awesome healing power of God. I agree with Jack Deere in *Surprised by the Power of the Spirit* when he contends that the real reason so many Christians do not believe in the healing power of God is "simply because they have not seen miracles in their present experience."[5] Before I witnessed these healings, I knew that Jesus healed in the Gospels, but I had not experienced His healing power today. But undeniable testimony of God's healing power happened right in front of me. So, both as a Christian and as a medical doctor, I began accepting the truth that God heals today, *naturally* and *supernaturally* or *miraculously*.

Understanding that God could and would heal in my medical practice through His Bible cure came slowly over the years as I saw God's Spirit work through the lives of so many patients in various and diverse situations. The ultimate revelation of the Bible cure came when I understood that God had a unique pathway of healing.

## GOD'S PATHWAY OF HEALING

1. In Jesus' healing miracles, one class of healing could be termed *instantaneous*. These were dramatic, sudden, instant miracles in which Jesus healed with supernatural spiritual power.

2. The second class of healing is *progressive healing*—people who were healed as they went. A healing process began at point A, but a time frame had to be played out to get to point B where the full manifestation of healing occurred.

In Daniel 10, the Bible cure reveals a mystery: while God answered Daniel's prayer instantly, there was a progressive manifestation of the answer over a twenty-one-day period of time. A supernatural being appears to Daniel and reveals to him that: " . . . for from the first day (מן־היות הראשון) that thou didst set thine heart to understand, and to chasten thyself before thy God, thy words were heard, and I am come for thy words" (Dan. 10:12). In other words, the moment Daniel prayed on that first day, God heard and answered his prayer. But twenty-one days passed before the answer to his prayer was manifested.

The moment we pray for healing, God hears and answers us. But the manifestation of our prayer's answer may take a number of days to be realized. A spiritual battle may well be taking place as it was with Daniel.

Later, in Daniel 10:14, the supernatural being revealed further that a vision received may be for a season or passage of days. God may supernaturally reveal a vision to you of your healing, but the healing will be manifested in a process over a season of time in your life.

An example of this Bible cure principle happening in the New Testament can be found in the story of Jesus' healing of the ten lepers (Luke 17). When they cried out from the roadside for their healing, Jesus instructed them to go at once and show themselves to the priests. The Greek text reads: καὶ ἐγένετο ἐν τῷ ὑπάγειν αὐτοὺς ἐκαθαρίσθησαν (Luke 17:14b). So we read, "As they went, they were cured. The Amplified Version translates the Greek this way: "And as they went they were cured and made clean." In other words, these lepers experienced a process of healing. As they went και εγενετο εν τω υπαγειν αυτοὺ, they were cured. As they obeyed Christ and did what He commanded, they encountered a passage of time that led to their healing.

This is similar to what Namaan had to do in the Old Covenant. (See 2 Kings 5:10.) While God gave him the assurance of his healing through Elisha, Namaan had to make his way to the Jordan and dip himself seven times in the waters. There was a process—a passage of time—that occurred before the full manifestation of his healing was evident.

The first remarkable revelation of the Bible cure that came to me in the practice of medicine while I was still a baby Christian was this: *God can heal both instantly and gradually.*

The manifestation of healing may occur instantaneously or it may manifest as a process.

## GOD'S PATHWAY OF HEALING

A SECOND AWESOME revelation from the Bible cure for me was this: *Healing anointing can flow through natural substances.* That was a tremendous revelation to me for the practice of medicine. If every healing came only through the supernatural, why would we need medicine? Why would we need to monitor blood pressure? Why would we need any kind of pill or even need doctors?

The Bible cure's pathway of healing is dramatically revealed in the ninth chapter of John where Jesus heals a blind man. Healing may be manifested instantaneously or as a process over a period of time. In God's pathway of healing, I discovered that God's healing may flow supernaturally, through natural substances, or through a combination of both!

In John 9:1–7, Jesus touched a blind man, but he wasn't healed instantly when Jesus touched him. As I really read that for the first time, it became a revelation to me. As a baby Christian, I thought that any time Jesus touched anybody, the power of God was so incredible that it just obliterated affliction immediately. But in John 9, Jesus touched the man, and then He gave him instructions to go and wash in the pool at Siloam. Jesus spat on the ground and made a clay ointment with His saliva, which He then applied to the blind man's eyes: ταῦτα εἰπὼν ἔπτυσεν χαμαὶ καὶ ἐποίησεν πηλὸν ἐκ τοῦ πτύσματος καὶ ἐπέχρισεν αὐτοῦ τὸν πηλὸν ἐπὶ τοὺς ὀφθαλμοὺς (John 9:6). As the blind man went to the pool and washed the mud from his eyes, he was healed.

---

### ἐπιχρίω — *"To anoint or apply an ointment"*

Ω The Bible cure is very specific in its use of language. The only place this Greek word ἐπιχρίω is found in the New Testament is in John 9:6. This word is from the vocabulary of the ancient Greek world of medicine. In fact, it is used by the Greek physician, Claudius Galen, in his medical writings, *Corpus Medicorum Graecorum*.[6] Galen resided in Rome, where he was the imperial physician attending Emperor Marcus Aurelius. He is called the father of experimental physiology.

So the Gospel writer John is using ancient medical terminology to refer to the way Jesus mixed the clay with His saliva to create a medicinal ointment for the blind man's eyes. John's ancient Greek text specifically points out that Jesus used natural substances in a medicinal way, combining them with supernatural, spiritual power to bring about healing to this blind man's eyes.

---

Jesus used both the natural and the spiritual in the blind man's healing (that is, healing anointing flowed through a natural substance). Similarly, in the Old Covenant, we see from the Bible cure that Namaan's healing from leprosy occurred as he used the natural substance of the Jordan's waters to wash himself.

Later in this book we will explore in depth both God's timetable and pathway of healing. But now, let's return to the mysteries hidden in the Bible cure from the Torah, or the first five books of the Old Testament. There we will see how God revealed, both in the Torah and in other places in the Old Covenant, how we could live in health through His commands and revelations of what to eat and how to live in the blessings of the Bible cure.

# 2

# God's Healing Secrets in the Old Covenant

IN THE OLD Covenant, the Bible cure reveals some insights about food and its effect upon our lives:

- Ways to avoid infectious diseases.
- Guidelines for temporary and permanent isolation of infection.
- Military hygiene and procedures that were used by the colonial army under George Washington.
- Reasons to avoid eating certain potentially harmful foods.
- Prohibitions against eating fatty foods.
- Avoidance of the consumption of blood.
- Healthy foods that can lengthen life and help prevent illnesses such as cancer, atherosclerosis, and cardiovascular diseases.
- God's pathway of healing through both the natural and supernatural.

The Jewish Tanach, named the Old Testament or Old Covenant by Christians, overflows with many revelations from God about hygiene, healthy foods, and the prophylaxis or prevention of diseases. As a medical doctor specializing in preventive medicine, I find the Old Covenant fascinating and intriguing. Throughout its ancient Hebrew text, one finds many unveiled secrets and mysteries concerning what we should eat, how to avoid contaminated and diseased objects, and what natural substances are used of God to effect healing and provide us with God's pathway of healing.

As we explore the Old Covenant together, I want to share some of the intriguing and life-giving revelations from the Bible cure that will guide you in a healthy lifestyle and point you in the direction of God's pathway of healing.

## ANCIENT ISRAEL AND MEDICINE

CURIOUSLY, AS A culture, the ancient Hebrews had very little interest in medicine or doctors. In fact, it wasn't until the Hellenistic period after 300 B.C. that medical science or physicians enjoyed any respect or prestige. T. A. Burkill, from the University of Rhodesia, remarks:

> Until well into the Hellenistic period physicians as such enjoyed little prestige, being ever suspected of impiety or charlatanism. Methods of therapy were fundamentally either magical or theurgical in character, and hygienic precautions were confined to such matters as cleansing a newborn infant with water, rubbing its body with salt, and swathing it with bands.[1]

The fact that the ancient Hebrews regarded medicine and physicians with suspicion makes the revelations in the Bible cure of the Old Covenant even more amazing. The insight that the ancient Jews looked askance at physicians is confirmed by the precise text of 2 Chronicles 16:12: "In the thirty-ninth year of his reign Asa was diseased in his feet, until his disease became very severe; yet in his disease he did not seek the

Lord, but relied on the physicians" (AMP). Apparently Asa waited until his disease became unmanageable before he consented to allow a physician to look at him. I do take a little comfort by noting in 1 Kings 15:23 that when reporting this incident, the writer dealt more charitably with physicians by simply reporting that Asa was diseased in his feet and not mentioning physicians at all!

---

### The Respect of Physicians and Medicine Among the Jews

Under the influence of Hellenism after Alexander the Greek conquered the known world in 333 B.C., Jewish scholars, influenced by Greek language and culture (Hellenism), translated the books of the Tanach (Old Covenant or Testament) and other revered writings known as the Apocrypha from Hebrew and Aramaic into Greek. This translation was known as the Septuagint (LXX). One of the books in the Septuagint reveals the emerging respect doctors were beginning to receive at the turn of the era compared to the ancient Hebrew suspicions of physicians. Ecclesiasticus 38:1–4 reads, "Honor the physician with the honor due him, according to your need of him, for the Lord created him; for healing comes from the Most High, and he will receive a gift from the king. The skill of the physician lifts up his head, and in the presence of great men he is admired. The Lord created medicines from the earth, and a sensible man will not despise them" (RSV).

---

The Hebrews did not seek to know more about anatomy, science, or the natural order as did their counterparts in the ancient civilizations of Egypt, Mesopotamia, or Greece. Quite the contrary. Anything that might be uncovered in the ancient Hebrew texts of the Bible had to come to them through divine, supernatural knowledge revealed by God. So what we shall unearth from the Old Covenant does not arise from human speculations on health and medicine but rather from God's particular Word to us about His pathway of healing for us—His creation. As Creator, God knows more about our bodies, His creation, than we could ever discover either through philosophy or science. God's knowledge of and care for our temples (physical bodies) is revealed in Psalm 139:13–16 (cf. 1 Cor. 3:16–19; 2 Cor. 6:16):

> For thou hast possessed my reins: thou hast covered me in my mother's womb. I will praise thee; for I am fearfully and wonderfully made: marvellous are thy works; and that my soul knoweth right well. My substance was not hid from thee, when I was made in secret, and curiously wrought in the lowest parts of the earth. Thine eyes did see my substance, yet being unperfect; and in thy book all my members were written, which in continuance were fashioned, when as yet there was none of them.

Since God created our bodies, He knows how they should be maintained and repaired. The Bible cure contains some incredible clues for preventing disease and healing afflicted bodies and souls.

## HEALTH AND HYGIENE

THE TORAH (PENTATEUCH), the first five books of the Bible, is also known as the Law. Within the Torah are three categories of Law—moral, health, and ceremonial. The Hebrews' righteousness was based on keeping the Law. Of course, no one could be righteous under the Law because it was impossible to keep the whole Law. Everyone has sinned and fallen short of God's righteousness (Rom. 3:23).

Under the New Covenant, Christians keep the moral law of the Torah, which we know as the Ten Commandments, but not in order to be righteous before God. We keep that law through the power of His Spirit, and we know that Christ is our righteousness. (See Zechariah 4:6; 1 Corinthians 1.) Jesus, by His Spirit, empowers us to keep the moral law. He came not to destroy the Law but to fulfill it (Matt. 5:17).

---

### תורה *Torah*

**א** *Torah* means "teaching or instruction." Because of Israel's constant disobedience, the prophets looked for a time when, once again, the law would go forth directly from God out of Jerusalem (Isa. 2:3). Then God Himself will teach and judge according to the law. In Isaiah 42:3–4, the prophet reveals that it will be the suffering servant's task to render judgment according to truth and to give forth a new teaching or law. His law will surpass the Mosaic law. It will not disagree with the old but build on it. Its scope will be universal.

Jeremiah sees the establishment of a New Covenant in which the law will be written on the heart (Jer. 31:33). Man will be able to obey God from his inner life outward. Then the true purpose of the law—to lead man into a fruitful, abundant life of fellowship with God—will be fully realized.[2]

---

The truth revealed in the Bible cure within the Old Covenant health laws has not ceased under the New Covenant. Our health is still protected by following the Old Testament health laws. Our righteousness, however, is not dependent on keeping the health and other laws, as it was for the Israelites. These truths still apply, and we are responsible for taking care of our bodies, which are now the temples of the Holy Spirit. The Bible cure unveils certain secrets about food and health that instruct us how to take care of our temples in the New Covenant.

## THE TRUTH ABOUT FAT

IN THE FIRST chapter, I laid a foundation for understanding that the Torah forbids the consumption of foods containing harmful fatty substances (חלב) that contain LDL saturated fats. Why does the Bible cure command us not to consume such fatty foods? Two specific prohibitions are found in the Torah:

> It shall be a perpetual statute for your generations throughout all your dwellings, that ye eat neither fat nor blood.
>
> —LEVITICUS 3:17

> Speak unto the children of Israel, saying, Ye shall eat no manner of fat, of ox, or of sheep, or of goat.
>
> —LEVITICUS 7:23

Why is this prohibition against fat so important for us? Over 53 percent of people in large industrialized countries die of heart disease. Heart disease is most commonly caused by fat deposits that build up in the arteries, often beginning in the teenage years. Symptoms range from angina (tightness or pressure in the chest), to severe pain associated with a heart attack, to congestive heart failure with fluid accumulation in the body. The following dietary steps, which are based on the Bible cure, will help a person to reduce fat intake and obey God's law for our own benefits.

Reduce your fat intake by:

- Eating lean beef no more than three to four times per month.

- Using only olive and canola oil.

- Consuming no meat at all three days per week. On those days eat only fruits and vegetables.

- Eating fish at least two or three times per week, preferably "cold-water" fish like salmon, cod, and herring.

Avoiding foods with saturated fats also provides protection against prostrate cancer. Prostate cancer is now the most common tumor in men who are nonsmokers. It will strike over a quarter million men yearly and kill over forty thousand men. The new blood test (PSA) should be done on all men over age fifty and on men under age fifty who have a family history of prostate cancer.

God promised in Exodus 23:25: "And ye shall serve the LORD your God, and he shall bless thy bread, and thy water; and I will take sickness away from the midst of thee." Notice that God takes away our sickness but His blessing first rests upon our choices of food. Certain foods contain God's healing substances.

All men should follow the eight steps listed below to help prevent prostate cancer from forming and to help cure it if the disease has been contracted:

1. *Decrease saturated fat.* Eat lean beef no more than three or four times a month. Avoid cheese and switch to skim milk. Red meat is especially linked to increased risk. Avoid mayonnaise, creamy salad dressings, and butter because of fatty acids (alpha linoleic acid). Use olive oil and canola oil.

2. *Antioxidants.* Get plenty of vitamins C, E, and beta carotene from yellow, orange, and dark green fruits and vegetables. Almonds (about ten per day) can supply vitamin E. Add these supplements: C (1,000 mg. twice daily); E (800 IU daily); beta carotene (30 mg., 50,000 IU daily).

3. *Calcium.* This can help decrease tumor formation and accumulation of a fatty acid that causes tumor formation (alpha linoleic acid). Get calcium from nonfat yogurt, nonfat cottage cheese, or skim milk. Add 1,000 milligrams of calcium (calcium carbonate) daily to your diet.

4. *Garlic.* The more garlic people have in their diet, the less their cancer incidence. Garlic can limit tumor growth markedly, kill cancer cells, and shrink tumors. Use a garlic press or take capsules daily that are equivalent to one clove of garlic. Take consistently.

5. *Vitamin D.* High levels of vitamin D can protect men from prostate cancer. Men in sunny climates have a lower incidence of prostate cancer. Sunlight helps the skin to produce vitamin D, but avoid

overexposure to the sun. Good sources of vitamin D can be found in skim milk and fish. Be careful with supplements. A dosage of 200 international units per day can be toxic. Get vitamin D from foods.

6. *Tea.* Compounds in green tea can inhibit tumor growth. Drink two cups per day. Lipton and other companies make green tea.

7. *Soy.* Soy products can limit the spread of cancer and can stop its early growth. Tofu and soy burgers are two sources for this protective food.

8. *Cumin.* This spice may prevent the development of prostate cancer. It can be used on vegetables and in various dishes.

## CLEANLINESS AND QUARANTINE

THE BIBLE CURE commanded the ancient Israelites to observe cleanliness and to quarantine disease long before science ever discovered the realities of infectious diseases.

The earliest mention of cleanliness in the Torah can be found in Exodus 19:10: "And the LORD said unto Moses, Go unto the people, and sanctify them to day and to morrow, and let them wash their clothes." Washing as a rite of purification, hygiene, and cleanliness was prescribed by the Law in reference to one's skin, clothing, housing, and food.

## CLEAN (טהר) AND UNCLEAN (טמא) ANIMALS

THE LISTS OF clean and unclean animals in Leviticus 11 and Deuteronomy 14 have a significance often ignored. Far from being a catalog of food taboos based on fad or fancy, these lists emphasize a fact not discovered until late in the last century and still not generally known: Animals carry diseases dangerous to man.

Five general groups are recognized—*mammals, birds,*

*reptiles, water animals,* and *insects*—though not in these precise terms.

1. *Mammals:* The clean, furred animals belong to one type only, whether domesticated or wild. They are known as ruminants, or animals that chew the cud, and are still our most important meat-producers. Some others are considered edible, but it was safer to have a simple rule—any clean mammal was both cloven-hoofed and a chewer of the cud. Those that were one or the other were ruled out, and three such animals are named: the hare, hyrax, and pig. The main purpose was probably to exclude the pig, now known to be the host for several serious human parasites. Pork is safe only when thoroughly cooked. Further, the pig is a scavenger and may spread other diseases mechanically.

2. *Birds:* Birds are so much more varied that they cannot be specifically classified. The forbidden kinds of birds are named; all others may be eaten. Some of these names are very difficult, with no help in the context of the language, and translations vary widely. But there is general agreement that the forbidden birds are the birds of prey—crows and other scavenging and carnivorous birds.

3. *Reptiles:* The list in Leviticus 11:29–30 is thought to consist mostly of reptiles, all of which are forbidden. In verse 42, a snake is banned: " . . . whatsoever goeth upon the belly."

4. *Water animals:* Although fish are not actually named in any list, they are included in the wider class of "everything in the waters" (Lev. 11:9). In fact, the qualification in this group is that the "clean" ones should have fins and scales. All crustaceans, shellfish, and the like are wisely excluded.

5. *Insects:* In spite of their great numbers, few kinds of insects are eaten, even in countries short of animal protein. Termites (white ants) may be locally useful, but the grasshopper family—easily recognized by the pair of jumping legs—is by far the most important. These are the only clean insects in the Mosaic law, described by the quaint but vivid phrase, " . . . which have legs above their feet, to leap withal upon the earth" (Lev. 11:21). Locusts are best termed "gregarious grasshoppers." They are wholly vegetarian and are useful food because of their high protein and calorie content. In warmer countries, locusts have been a standard food since early times, and it is likely that they were eaten regularly on the desert march.[3]

Certain living creatures were pronounced clean (טהר) or unclean (טמא). The Hebrew text for the Bible cure reads: להבדיל בין הטמא ובין הטהר. Translated, it states: "To make a difference between the *unclean* and the *clean . . .*" (Lev. 11:47, emphasis added). The clean animals could be eaten while the prohibition was against eating what was unclean. The dead bodies of humans and animals were pronounced unclean and not to be touched. If they were, then one was unclean until ceremonial washing was done as commanded. Here is a sampling of some of those passages in the Levitical cure referring to that which is unclean:

> Or if a soul touch any unclean thing, whether it be a carcase of an unclean beast, or a carcase of unclean cattle, or the carcase of unclean creeping things, and if it be hidden from him; he also shall be unclean, and guilty.
>
> —LEVITICUS 5:2

> Nevertheless these shall ye not eat of them that chew the cud, or of them that divide the hoof: as the camel, because he cheweth the cud, but divideth not the hoof; he is unclean unto you.
>
> —LEVITICUS 11:4

This is the law of the beasts, and of the fowl, and of every living creature that moveth in the waters, and of every creature that creepeth upon the earth: To make a difference between the unclean and the clean, and between the beast that may be eaten and the beast that may not be eaten.

—LEVITICUS 11:46–47

And upon whatsoever any of them, when they are dead, doth fall, it shall be unclean; whether it be any vessel of wood, or raiment, or skin, or sack, whatsoever vessel it be, wherein any work is done, it must be put into water, and it shall be unclean until the even; so it shall be cleansed.

—LEVITICUS 11:32

And the priest shall look on the plague in the skin of the flesh: and when the hair in the plague is turned white, and the plague in sight be deeper than the skin of his flesh, it is a plague of leprosy: and the priest shall look on him, and pronounce him unclean.

—LEVITICUS 13:3

These shall ye eat of all that are in the waters: whatsoever hath fins and scales in the waters, in the seas, and in the rivers, them shall ye eat. And all that have not fins and scales in the seas, and in the rivers, of all that move in the waters, and of any living thing which is in the waters, they shall be an abomination unto you . . . Whatsoever hath no fins nor scales in the waters, that shall be an abomination unto you.

—LEVITICUS 11:9–10, 12

And the swine, though he divide the hoof, and be cloven-footed, yet he cheweth not the cud; he is unclean to you.

—LEVITICUS 11:7

Notice that certain types of animals were unclean to eat, particularly swine and seafood such as shrimp or oysters that did not have scales. Why? The Bible cure revealed the potentially unhealthy (unclean) attributes of these meats centuries before science uncovered that pork could carry the deadly trichinosis infection and that shrimp or shellfish retain heavy metals—mercury or lead—in their flesh.

Those with infectious diseases such as leprosy were quarantined to protect the general population from contracting these diseases. Earlier I mentioned the Torah's prohibition against eating fat or blood (Lev. 7:26). This prohibition against consuming blood concurs with our present medical knowledge that blood can be a vehicle for spreading infectious diseases. F. H. Garrison, in his classic study on medical history, writes:

> The ancient Hebrews were in fact the founders of prophylaxis, and the high priests were true medical police. They had a definite cure of ritual hygiene and cult cleanliness. . . . The Book of Leviticus contains the sternest mandates in regard to touching unclean objects, the proper food to be eaten, the purifying of women after childbirth, the hygiene of the menstrual period, the abomination of sexual perversions, and the prevention of contagious diseases. In the remarkable chapter on the diagnosis and prevention of leprosy, gonorrhea, and leukorrhea (Leviticus XIII:XV), the most definite common-sense directions are given in regard to segregation, disinfection (even to the point of scraping the walls of the house or destroying it completely), and the old Mosaic rite to incineration of the patient's garments and other fomites.[4]

A key principle of medicine can be unearthed in the study of the Bible cure: The rights of an individual are limited when one's health or conduct endangers the health of the corporate society. This notion of corporate personality also is reflected in the New Covenant. Paul writes, "That there should be no schism in the body; but that the members should have the same care one for another. And whether one member suffer, all the members suffer with it; or one member be honoured, all the members rejoice with it" (1 Cor. 12:25–26). The Bible cure not only provided for the health and healing of the individual but also for the corporate whole as well.

The Bible cure's rules of hygiene found in the Torah were so effective that the colonial army under General George Washington followed them! General Washington ordered the army under General McDougall's command to follow the hygiene prescribed in the Deuteronomic cure as military rules for hygiene and policing the camps. The Bible cure that Washington ordered as a military procedure states:

> If there be among you any man, that is not clean by reason of uncleanness that chanceth him by night, then shall he go abroad out of the camp, he shall not come within the camp: But it shall be, when evening cometh on, he shall wash himself with water: and when the sun is down, he shall come into the camp again. Thou shalt have a place also without the camp, whither thou shalt go forth abroad: And thou shalt have a paddle upon thy weapon; and it shall be, when thou wilt ease thyself abroad, thou shalt dig therewith, and shalt turn back and cover that which cometh from thee: For the Lord thy God walketh in the midst of thy camp, to deliver thee, and to give up thine enemies before thee; therefore shall thy camp be holy: that he see no unclean thing in thee, and turn away from thee.
> —Deuteronomy 23:10–14

General Washington specifically observed:

> In the History of these People, the soldiers must admire the singular attention that was paid to the Rules of Cleanliness. They were obliged to wash their Hands two or three Times a Day. Foul garments were counted abominable: every Thing that was polluted or dirty was absolutely Forbidden: and such Persons as had Sores or Diseases in their skin were turned out of the Camp. The utmost pains were taken to keep the Air in which they breathed, free from infection. They were commanded to

have a place without the Camp, whither they should go, and have a paddle with which they should dig so that when they went abroad to ease themselves they might turn back and cover that which came from them.[5]

In ancient times, the Bible cure helped both priests and ordinary people to recognize diseases and inhibit their spread. As we shall discover in the following pages, the foods eaten in the kosher diets prescribed by the Torah helped to prevent disease while maintaining health and longevity. The Bible cure also observed such emotional illnesses as depression and recognized the curative affects of music in the treatment of depressive illness. (See 1 Samuel 16:23.) Today it is a well-accepted medical practice to integrate music into the treatment of patients with chronic or mental illnesses.

Many of the foods found in the Old Covenant and prescribed by the dietary laws can be observed today in what we describe as the Mediterranean Diet, which I will detail in the next chapter. Now let's turn our attention to some of the revelations contained in the Bible cure from the New Covenant.

## JESUS, THE GREAT PHYSICIAN

THE BIBLE CURE under the Old Covenant revealed many natural ways that God has actually built into the fabric of creation, particularly through food and hygiene, to help us walk in our pathway of healing. Remember that our pathway of healing contains both natural and supernatural ways that God heals. Jesus, as the Great Physician, focused much of His early ministry on two activities—healing and teaching.

The fact that He was continually moved by compassion to heal points us to this reality from the Bible cure: Jesus wills that we be in good health and be healed from all diseases. This truth is dramatically demonstrated when Jesus encounters a leper:

> And there came a leper to him, beseeching him, and kneeling down to him, and saying unto him, If thou wilt, thou canst

make me clean. And Jesus, moved with compassion, put forth his hand, and touched him, and saith unto him, *I will;* be thou clean. And as soon as he had spoken, immediately the leprosy departed from him, and he was cleansed.

—MARK 1:40–42, EMPHASIS ADDED

Jesus regarded Himself as a physician of body *and* soul:

But when Jesus heard that, he said unto them, They that be whole need not a physician, but they that are sick.

—MATTHEW 9:12

When Jesus heard it, he saith unto them, They that are whole have no need of the physician, but they that are sick: I came not to call the righteous, but sinners to repentance.

—MARK 2:17

And he said unto them, Ye will surely say unto me this proverb, Physician, heal thyself: whatsoever we have heard done in Capernaum, do also here in thy country.

—LUKE 4:23

In fact, Jesus is the Messiah seen prophetically in Jeremiah 8:22: "Is there no balm in Gilead; is there no physician there? Why then is not the health of the daughter of my people recovered?"

The ministry of Jesus has, as a primary focus, the restoring of health to diseased bodies and tormented souls. Everywhere Jesus traveled in the Gospels, He acted like the Great Physician. In the four Gospels there are forty-one distinct pericopes of physical and mental healing (with a total of seventy-two accounts in all, counting all duplications). In many stories, not just one person but multitudes were healed.

## Σώζω — *Heal, Save, and Make Whole*

Ω In Greek, there is a symbiotic connection between salvation and healing. One is saved from sin and hell for righteousness and eternal life. But σωζω also refers to curing from illness. A physical life is healed from disease. (See Acts 4:9; 14:9; John 11:12; James 5:15.) In resurrection, the body is raised and changed from mortality to immortality. In the Gospels, the healings of Jesus use σώζω sixteen times to refer to physical and mental healing. Often faith is linked to healing, and the whole person is referred to as being saved. (See Matthew 8:25; Luke 7:50.)[6]

In the first chapter, I detailed some important truths about the Bible cure that can be learned from Jesus' ministry and teaching. These truths I call the *pathway of healing*. I want to explore the pathway of healing now with specificity.

## THE BIBLE CURE'S PATHWAY OF HEALING

IT'S WONDERFUL TO read in the Gospels about Jesus' miraculous healings. But some may wonder if Jesus is still the Great Physician. Hebrews 13:8 reveals, "Jesus Christ the same yesterday, and to day, and for ever." That means that the Messiah who healed two thousand years ago still heals today.

When Jesus walked the hills of Palestine, sophisticated medicine did not exist. No intricate equipment, computers, or medical labs existed. However, people were healed supernaturally. They also received healing in other ways through God's pathway of healing.

For example, the ten lepers were healed "as they went." The blind man was healed as Jesus applied mud and saliva to his eyes.

Healings occur today in our modern society just as they did in the ancient biblical world. Healings happen both through the healing anointing on natural medicine and through the supernatural move of God's healing power through the Holy Spirit.

I want to summarize for you the principles of the Bible cure's pathway of healing.

1. *God has a specific pathway of healing just for you.*

While the testimony of others can encourage you, their pathway may not be yours. Jesus said to the leper in Luke 17, "Go thy way (αναστα πορευου)" (Luke 17:19). *Way* can be translated as "journey or life direction."

In other words, Jesus is not specifying just any pathway or journey, but the specific and particular way that one leper must go in order to walk in his healing. Christ desires for you to walk in your pathway of healing—not in someone else's.

Let's take another example. Elisha sent his messenger to tell Namaan, "Go, wash yourself seven times in the Jordan" (2 Kings 5:10, NIV). Not everyone with leprosy should go wash in the Jordan, only Namaan. That was his specific pathway of healing from God.

2. *Pray and seek God for your pathway of healing.*

Because God is an infinite God, He possesses infinite ways to heal. His possibilities for your healing are unlimited by time or method. Since, as your Creator, He knows every molecule in your being, God knows exactly what your Bible cure is. (See Psalm 139:13–16.) So seek Him for your pathway. James writes, "Is anyone among you sick? Let him call for the elders of the church, and let them pray . . . " (James 5:14, NAS). Are you praying and seeking God for your Bible cure—your specific and particular pathway of healing?

3. *God uses the natural and the supernatural to heal.*

Don't limit God to your expectations of how He will heal you. As a Christian physician, I see people make this mistake over and over again. They come to me with their minds already made up on how they expect God to bring about their

31

healing. In doing so, they limit God and may completely miss their Bible cure.

Remember, Jesus used clay and saliva to heal the blind man in John 9. In Matthew 9, He simply touched the eyes of two blind men. In Mark 8, Jesus spat on a blind man's eyes and asked him if he saw anything. When the man could only see men who looked like trees walking, Jesus then put His hands on the man's eyes, and he recovered.

In each instance, the same illness—blindness—was healed in different ways. You may have the same kind of cancer as someone else that you know, but their Bible cure could be very different from yours. Seek God's pathway of healing for you. Don't seek someone else's pathway.

4. *Your healing may be instantaneous—or a process.*

You may wish to be healed instantly. The healing manifestation may occur over a period of time. Remember, God says that His ways are not our ways, and His thoughts are not our thoughts (Isa. 55:8–9). Recall also Daniel chapter 10: there may be a great battle being fought in the heavenlies for your healing to manifest.

Let's turn our attention to some wonderful clues to the Bible cure that are unveiled in the writings of the ancient physician, Luke.

## LUKE, THE PHYSICIAN

BEFORE LOOKING AT some specific foods that are revealed in the Bible cure that have the ability to maintain health and prevent disease, we can briefly explore two very interesting insights into the Bible cure.

First, the Gospel writer Luke was a doctor who used specific medical language to describe Jesus' ministry and some of the events in the Book of Acts. Exciting insights about healing can be uncovered in the Greek texts written by Luke, the beloved physician. (See Colossians 4:14.)

Second, we shall briefly mention the Apocrypha and

Talmud as ancient texts that supplement and further augment the Bible cure.

Luke resided in Antioch, one of the great cities of the Roman empire on the commercial trade routes between Asia Minor and Africa. Luke was educated in and exposed to the best medical knowledge of his day. Luke used Greek medical terminology, which indicated that he was well acquainted with the diseases and medical conditions that he described. In fact, "he used language only an educated physician would use; language which shared the common medical idiom of the period. The phraseology consistently exhibits similarities of structure, style, and choice of words with those found in the works of Hippocrates, Aretaeus, Dioscorides, and Galen. This analysis strongly supports the view that Saint Luke was a physician well educated in the Greek medical tradition."[7]

In Luke's writings, the Bible cure unveils some very interesting revelations. Scholars have long noted the parallels among the synoptic Gospels—Matthew, Mark, and Luke. These first three Gospels have many overlapping texts that have identical or almost identical wording. This has led some scholars to conclude that the Book of Mark was the earliest Gospel and served as the chronological outline for both Matthew and Luke, which follow.

Without further discussion of this theory, we can observe that when Luke does agree textually with Matthew and Mark, he often uses his own medical language to describe Jesus' healing miracles instead of following the terms of Matthew or Mark. His use of Greek medical terminology leads us to discover interesting insights from the Bible cure.

---

### Ὑγιαίνω—Be Healthy, Sound

**Ω** In secular Greek, ὑγιαίνω refers to being healthy or whole. Healing is viewed as an esteemed craft, and the health of both soul and body is important. The Septuagint speaks of health forty-one times and views ὑγιαίνω as a divine gift. In the New Testament, ὑγιαίνω is used in the Gospels in reference to Jesus as victor over sin and suffering. He restores health by His word. (See Matthew 12:13; Mark 5:34; Luke 5:31; John 5:9). Making the whole person healthy, Jesus liberates one for a new life that embraces the physical body (John 7:23). He transmits His power to heal, or to make whole, to the apostles (Acts 4:10).[8]

---

*Be healthy* (ὑγιαίνω). "And Jesus answering said unto them, They that are whole (ὑγιαίνω) need not a physician (ἰατρός) but they that are sick" (Luke 5:31). Matthew 9:12 and Mark 2:17 describe "they that are whole" as "strong" (ἰσχύοντες), not "healthy" (ὑγιαίνω).

The Bible cure reveals that Jesus has a deep compassion for healing those who are sick. We may even conjecture that beyond healing, the Great Physician, Jesus, has a primary concern for people's health! Why? Because healthy people can witness energetically of Jesus Christ as Lord and Savior. They have the energy and strength to work in God's kingdom, obediently doing His will. Healthy people can minister to and care for those who are sick, poor, and disadvantaged. What a poor witness I would be as a physician if my patients found me to be in poor health because I did not take care of the temple that the Word created for me and is sustained by His Spirit!

*The physican's therapy* (θεραπεία). Luke used some Greek medical terms that are found nowhere else in the New Testament. One such term is θεραπεία, from which we get the word "therapy." So Luke writes:

> And the people, when they knew it, followed him: and
> he received them, and spake unto them of the kingdom

of God, and healed them that had need of healing
[therapy—θεραπεία].

—Luke 9:11

*Therapy* refers to healing, restoring to health, and doing medical procedures that will effect healing. As the Great Physician, Jesus employed both the supernatural and natural means given to Him by the Father to restore sight to the blind, healing to the leper, and health to the sick in body and soul. From Luke's perspective, we may presume that Jesus acted and healed like a physician—not like a magician or charlatan. Jesus' healing was not superstitious or occult as the Pharisees and religious leaders accused. (See Matthew 9:34.) Rather, Jesus was a vessel of God's creative and restorative power to take broken creatures and heal them through the will and miracle-working power of their Creator.

## ᾿Ιάομαι —*Heal or Cure*

Ω The noun ἰατρός is translated "physician." The physician is the object, vessel, or instrument of healing. A person is healed or cured from a physical illness or delivered from ills of many kinds. Some Jews in Jesus' day believed illness to be caused by sin in one's life. So healing (ἰάομαι) would also include being cured of the wound caused in one's soul by sin.[9]

*Jesus heals all our diseases.* Luke witnessed Jesus heal physical afflictions with definite somatic symptoms that Luke described with medical precision. Much more than the other Gospel writers, Luke the physician uses the word ἰάομαι, which specifically means "to heal or cure in a medical sense," and comes from the Greek word ἰατρός meaning "physician." The English words *iatrogenic* and *pediatrics* are derived from this word. Even more amazing is that the Greek noun for healing is ἴασις, which is only found twice in the New Testament (Luke 13:32 and Acts 4:22). So Luke alone uses the technical, medical term for healing (ἴασις) in the New Testament!

*Jesus is the Great Physician.* There is only one reference in the Gospels in which Jesus refers to Himself as a physician:

> Ye will surely say unto me this proverb, Physician (Ἰατρέ), heal thyself: whatsoever we have heard done in Capernaum, do also here in thy country. And he said, Verily I say unto you, No prophet is accepted in his own country." Jesus did not shy away from being seen as a physician by those around Him. He acknowledged both the role and the attacks that went with it.
>
> —LUKE 4:23–24

The Bible cure as revealed in Luke's writings leads us to some interesting observations and discoveries. In summary:

- The Bible cure unveils an ancient understanding and appreciation for medicine and medical treatment, confirming in the New Covenant and in the Old that God uses both the natural and the supernatural to heal.

- Jesus had compassion for those with all diseases—physical and mental. And He healed all diseases.

- Christ's ministry placed an emphasis and priority on healing the physical as well as the spiritual. Jesus wills to save (σῴζω) and heal (σῴζω) body, soul, and spirit.

- Luke portrays Jesus, the Great Physician, as one who treated the sick as a physician, using the most profound natural skill and supernatural gifts to usher people into their specific pathways of healing.

# 3

# God's Principles That Reveal Your Pathway to Healing

THE BIBLE CURE has revealed six specific principles for iden-
tifying your particular pathway of healing. In your pathway
of healing, God may supernaturally and instantaneously heal
you, or you may experience a process that combines His
supernatural power and wisdom with specific actions necessary for you to take in the natural to obtain your healing.
These actions could even include surgery, therapy, medication, or nutrition, either separately or in combination with one
another. The Holy Spirit will use both Old and New Covenant
revelation from the Bible to direct you through your pathway
of healing.

While there is an order to these principles, God's Spirit may
choose to use these principles in overlapping ways to move
you toward your specific Bible cure. The experience and
knowledge of others may help and encourage you. But
another person's pathway, even if they have had similar
symptoms or diagnosis, may not be God's pathway for you.
These Bible-cure principles will enable you to walk through

God's pathway of healing for you.

One of the first things I advise a patient who is seeking God for a Bible cure is the importance of being informed about the wiles of the devil. Paul gives these instructions: "Lest Satan should get an advantage of us: for we are not ignorant of his devices. . . . Put on the whole armour of God, that ye may be able to stand against the wiles of the devil" (2 Cor. 2:11; Eph. 6:11). The first thing a person must ask is: "What is it that has attacked me?"

Medicine approaches a physical problem in much the same way through diagnosing the problem afflicting a person's body. So when Satan attacks our bodies, part of that attack can be in the natural or physical realm. Through medicine, God has given us certain skills and techniques for diagnosing the natural schemes and devices that Satan may be using to attack our bodies.

When a person is physically ill, the devil may indeed be attacking—and there also may be other causes for that illness. For example, I sometimes explain to patients that they may have come out from under the umbrella of protection that God has placed over His children. (See Job 1:10.) When we are disobedient or ignorant of God's will for our lives, we can remove ourselves from God's hand of protection. Then we become vulnerable to the devil's attacks.

We may be disobedient by eating foods that are unhealthy for us, such as foods high in saturated fats. Or we may not be exercising and staying physically fit. Perhaps we have allowed sin, unforgiveness, worry, cares, or stress to work their destructive attacks on our bodies. Out from under God's umbrella of protection, we are exposed to the attacks of darkness from the "prince of the air" (Eph. 2:2). So we may diagnose the physical illness, but we also need spiritual insight to understand that a physical attack on our bodies comes from the realm of darkness. Medical diagnosis is not enough in understanding our illness. We also must not be ignorant of the devices of the devil.

It is important to realize that the righteous, although under the umbrella of God's protection, can suffer. In other words, we can be attacked. The Bible says, "Many are the afflictions of the righteous: but the LORD delivereth him out of them all" (Ps. 34:19). We may not understand why some of the afflictions beset us. Yet, a person may simply be such a threat to the kingdom of darkness that Satan attacks with all his devices. I believe, however, that the Christian who walks under God's umbrella of protection has the advantage of revelation knowledge and thus can overcome any attack of the enemy. "Greater is he [the Holy Spirit] that is in you, than he [Satan] that is in the world" (1 John 4:4).

When you have identified what the attack is, then you are ready to apply the principles of the Bible cure in order to uncover God's pathway of healing for you. Let's examine each principle of the Bible cure.

When a medical doctor has made a diagnosis, he goes by a protocol or set of rules compiled by experts in medicine and based on the best natural consensus of knowledge that they have acquired. But the Bible cure instructs us that God's ways are not our ways and His thoughts are not our thoughts (Isa. 55:8–9). God's pathway of healing does not always follow the strict protocols of medicine. His wisdom and knowledge far exceed anything that finite knowledge, experience, or research in the field of medicine has learned. The Bible cure does not ask what the doctor and medicine want us to do in order to find healing. The definitive question asked by the Bible cure is: *What does God want me to do?*

Does God want me simply to stand on His Word in faith as I confess that by His stripes I have been healed? Does God want to combine His supernatural healing power with natural substances and medical treatment? The anointing of God can flow through natural substances (John 9:1–7). Natural substances may include medicine, surgery, medication, a chemical in a plant, or a combination of many natural elements that God ordains to use in a specific person's pathway of healing.

In Philippians 4:6 we are instructed, "Be careful for nothing." In other words, we are not to fear or be anxious about anything. In order to seek God in prayer for our pathway of healing, the Bible cure insists that we not worry—

*have no anxiety about anything.* How is this possible? This brings us to this first essential principle of the Bible cure:

## PRINCIPLE #1 — CAST YOUR CARES ON THE LORD

FEAR, ANXIETY, AND worry can hinder your prayers seeking the Spirit's guidance for your pathway of healing. The Bible cure reveals how to be set free from fear:

> Casting the whole of your care—all your anxieties, all your worries, all your concerns, once and for all—on Him; for He cares for you affectionately, and cares about you watchfully.
>
> —1 PETER 5:7, AMP

So often I see patients bound and consumed by anxiety and fear. They have observed physical symptoms in their bodies, and they are worried and anxious about the negative diagnosis they have been given by a doctor. Fear—the enemy they must overcome—is counterproductive to both their faith and prayers. Faith is a certainty of those things hoped for and evidence of things not yet seen (Heb. 11:1).

If you are facing such worries and fears, I want to reassure you that through Christ's stripes you have been healed. When I have patients who are fearful, I tell them about other patients whom God has healed. I say, "You have to cast your anxieties and cares upon God. You must cast your worries upon the Lord *once and for all!"*

I might have a patient with abdominal pain pray these words:

> I cast my fear about this pain in my abdomen *once and for all* upon You, Lord Jesus. Now here it is; I am giving it to You, Father. I know that You love and care for me. Your perfect love casts out every fear in me. In Jesus' name and by His stripes, I am healed. Amen.

I also warn my patient that the fear is very likely to attack again within a day or two after we have prayed. So I tell him *not* to pray the same prayer about fear again. Instead, I explain that the devil is attacking his mind with fear and his prayer should now be directed toward the devil. I remind him that he has already cast his cares, fears, and worries upon the Lord *once and for all!* He doesn't need to do that again. Now he must address a rebuke to the devil, saying, "Satan, I have cast anxiety about that pain in my abdomen on my heavenly Father, just as He told me to do. He would not tell me to cast my cares upon Him unless it is something I am capable of doing. Therefore, Satan, I take authority over you, and I command you to stop attacking my mind with fearful thoughts."

Satan may return again a few days later with the same recurring attack of fear. Again, I remind my patients that they must not cast their cares on the Lord again. He has already cast out their fears with His perfect love (1 John 4:18). After they rebuke the devil two or three times and bind the attacks upon their minds, the attacking fearful thoughts cease; my patients then find the peace that passes all understanding through Christ Jesus. I know that this principle of *casting your cares on the Lord* sets people free to pray and petition God for their Bible cure. It also releases their faith.

## PRINCIPLE #2 — PRAY AND PETITION GOD FOR YOUR PATHWAY OF HEALING

LET'S RETURN TO Philippians 4:6 where we read: "Do not fret or have any anxiety about anything" (AMP). When my patients have cast their cares upon God so that those anxieties are not hindering their prayer, then they are ready to pray and petition God according to the rest of verses 6 and 7:

> ...but in every thing by prayer and supplication with thanksgiving let your requests be made known unto God. And the peace of God, which passeth all understanding, shall keep your hearts and minds through Christ Jesus.

A *petition* is a definite request. When a patient has all the diagnostic information about his illness that is available, is not ignorant of the schemes and devices of the devil, and has cast all his cares on the Lord, then he is equipped to pray specifically and to petition God concerning his Bible cure.

One patient in his early twenties came to me with a genetic disease called neurofibromatosis. This was a rare disease you study about in medical school for a few hours and then go on because it is likely you will seldom even see a patient with this disease in the course of your medical practice. This disease was decimating the patient's family. The disorder affects about one in fifty thousand people, causing tumors to form on nerves, skin, and internal organs, which at times can become life-threatening. There is no known cure for neurofibromatosis. This man did not want to die from this disease like so many in his immediate family—his father and brother had already died, and his sister was near death. He told me that God had instructed him to come to me. We went over all the information we had about the disease and its attack on his body. Casting all fear on the Lord, we prepared to pray for his pathway of healing.

"Dr. Cherry," he said. "I don't want to die a young man. This disease is wiping out my family. I need your help."

In the natural as a physician, I was frustrated. I knew that there was no known treatment or cure medically for this disease. When I finished with his exam, I went into my office and started praying, "God, what is it that this man needs to know? He already has all the information about his disease that medicine can give him. What can I do to help him?"

The Lord led me to look at *Cecil's Textbook of Medicine.* I looked up the description of *neurofibromatosis* in this text. The Holy Spirit directed me to read this medical description to my patient and to tell him what caused the disease. I thought that he had all the information he needed in order for us to pray. But God knew that he needed something more than what he already knew. So I obeyed the Lord and read the description of this disease to him. The description mentioned that the end of chromosome 17 was genetically defective in this disease. When I read to him the specific cause of his disease, tears began to stream down this man's cheeks.

"That's what I came here for and why God told me to see you," he said. "I have been asking doctors for years what caused my disease, and none of them ever told me. Now that I know the specific cause—the defect in chromosome 17—I can pray for my healing." He continued by stating, "I don't want to die an early death. I want to serve God. There is much God wants me to do."

God had put in this man's spirit to pray specifically for his pathway of healing. We prayed together that the defect of chromosome 17 not be expressed in his body in the form of neurofibroma tumors.

I said, "You and I have agreed together in prayer that this defect will not be expressed in your body. Every day I want you to speak to that gene in chromosome 17, telling it to be normal and commanding it to be healed in Jesus' name." That was over five years ago; today that man is enjoying good health and serving God. He had prayed and petitioned God specifically for his Bible cure, and God had answered his prayer.

## PRINCIPLE #3 — TEST YOUR OPTIONS BY THE SPIRIT OF GOD

AS WE PRAY and petition God to reveal His Bible cure for us, we must let the Holy Spirit reveal our options and check or stop any choices that He does not desire. In Colossians 3:15, Paul writes, "Let the peace of God rule in your hearts." The Amplified Version expands our understanding of this verse by indicating that the peace of God acts as an umpire in our hearts: "Let the peace...from the Christ...act as an umpire continually...deciding and settling with finality all questions that arise in your minds." We have to ask the Holy Spirit to act as an umpire to help us decide and settle with finality the options that are before us so that His peace will rule in our hearts. The Spirit of God helps us sort through our options and decisions—He umpires our choices—until we reach a choice that brings complete peace in our lives. Until the Bible cure is revealed completely, we will have turmoil and indecision in our hearts.

At the same time that I am presenting and praying through with a patient all the options of his or her pathway of healing, I am testing those options as well. We must test each option before us and ask, "Is this what God's Spirit wants us to do?" When an option is not right, we should ask the Holy Spirit to put a check in our spirits, and to give us turmoil rather than peace in our hearts. We read in Acts 16:6, "Now when they had gone throughout Phrygia and the region of Galatia, and were *forbidden of the Holy Ghost* to preach the word in Asia..." From this we can learn that the Holy Spirit closes the door on certain options in our lives. In our hearts He checks us from making a certain decision or from going in a particular direction. There is a constraint of the Holy Spirit as well as peace from the Holy Spirit. We test our understanding of the Spirit's leading by asking, "Is this Jesus? Is this what God wants?" As God's Spirit acts as an umpire in our hearts, His leading will help us to experience His peace about the "open door" options we find and will help us to recognize turmoil and confusion as detrimental options to our healing.

For example, if a patient has cancer, she may be faced with many choices—radiation, chemotherapy, surgery, or other medical procedures. Should she not do any of these—or a combination of things? How many sessions of radiation or chemotherapy should she undergo if there is no check in the progress of her illness? Or does she simply stand in faith and wait while continuing to build up her immune system through good nutrition?

Often I will say to a patient, "The reason you are here is to find out if you have done all and now need to stand firm and in the peace of God."

I have seen so many Christians in turmoil running to and fro from clinics all throughout Europe, the Caribbean, or Mexico trying desperately to force a miracle cure instead of standing firm in the Lord, knowing that in His blood alone is the Bible cure for their lives. After testing all the options, the Holy Spirit will give us peace about those He desires us to pursue, and we can stand firm in His leading for our pathway of healing.

## PRINCIPLE #4—SPEAK TO YOUR MOUNTAIN

NOW WE ARE ready to speak to the mountain. Instead of just praying, petitioning, and testing, we must go further in our walk with God. Jesus taught us to speak to our mountain and command that illness to be removed:

> For verily I say unto you, That whosoever shall say unto this mountain, Be thou removed, and be thou cast into the sea; and shall not doubt in his heart, but shall believe that those things which he saith shall come to pass; he shall have whatsoever he saith. Therefore I say unto you, What things soever ye desire, when ye pray, believe that ye receive them, and ye shall have them.
>
> —MARK 11:23–24

As we follow the first three principles, by the time we reach this point we know what the devil's scheme…what the mountain…is. That mountain may be ovarian cancer, a blocked artery, or a tumor in the colon. Whatever it is, speak to it.

How do we speak to our mountain? If we are speaking to a blocked artery, we speak to that blockage to be absorbed and to regress. We speak to the platelets not to clot on that roughened plaque in the artery, which could form a blood clot causing a heart attack or stroke. In other words, we speak specifically and directly to our mountain because we now know what we face, what to pray, what actions the Holy Spirit does and does not want us to take, and how to let God's peace rule in our hearts concerning the options the Spirit has led us to choose.

When we speak to our mountain, we pray specifically about what the Holy Spirit has revealed to us. Instead of praying, "God, heal my body," we now pray, "God, I am praying that the plaque formation—this scheme and device of the enemy—regress, that the cholesterol be reabsorbed, and that there will be no platelets that can stick or bind to the plaque and obstruct the flow of blood. Your Word tells me that life is in the blood."

Let me give you another example. Suppose a patient knows that he has a melanoma in the advanced stages of the disease. A malignant melanoma is a type of skin cancer that can spread rapidly throughout the body when undetected and untreated. How would a person speak to this mountain specifically? He should pray: "Father, the work of darkness of melanoma has attacked my body. These cells of cancerous melanoma have divided abnormally in my body and have spread to my lymph nodes and vital organs. I know that You, God, have created within my body an immune system with cells designed and created by You to attack and destroy these abnormal cells. Therefore, Father, my petition and prayer before Your throne, pleading the blood of Jesus Christ, is that my immune system be activated. Lord, I say to my immune system, 'Rise up, attack any abnormal cells, and rid my entire body of this melanoma.' In addition, Father, I ask that the Holy Spirit continue to guide me to truth as to everything I need to do in the natural to enhance and strengthen my immune system."

So many times I have seen what medicine calls "spontaneous remission"—*I call it a healing by the power of God*—occur when a patient speaks to the mountain. Let me affirm that a remission lasting the rest of a person's life is more than a medical mystery; *it's the Bible cure!*

## PRINCIPLE #5 — PERSIST AND STAND FIRM IN YOUR BIBLE CURE

ONCE THE HOLY Spirit has revealed to you the steps to take in the Bible cure for your pathway of healing, giving you peace, and you have spoken to the mountain, then you have *done all* and must stand firm in the Lord.

In the tenth chapter of Daniel we see how Daniel persisted in prayer and stood firm in the Lord. A patient may not see immediate improvement or healing in his or her situation. I say to that person: "The reason you are going through this is because of the great battle that is occurring in the heavenlies. The powers and principalities of darkness are warring against your healing. In your physical body, you are feeling, sensing, and experiencing the violence of this spiritual battle. You are a threat to the devil and the kingdom of darkness. But when you presented your petition to God, your prayer was answered that first day. Now you are facing a time in which you must persist and stand firm believing for your Bible cure." I further explain that Daniel had to wait twenty-one days while God sent the archangel Michael to battle the forces of darkness and bring the full answer to Daniel's prayer. We too need to stand firm as Daniel did and persist in prayer as the widow did in her requests to the unjust judge in Luke:

> And he spake a parable unto them to this end, that men ought always to pray, and not to faint; saying, There was in a city a judge, which feared not God, neither regarded man: and there was a widow in that city; and she came unto him, saying, Avenge me of mine adversary. And he would not for a while: but afterwards he said within himself, Though I fear not God, nor regard man; yet because this widow troubleth me, I will avenge her, lest by her continual coming she weary me. And the Lord said, Hear what the unjust judge saith. And shall not God avenge his own elect, which cry day and night unto him, though he bear long with them? I tell you that he will avenge them speedily. Nevertheless when the Son of man cometh, shall he find faith on the earth?
>
> —LUKE 18:1–8

Faith—trusting God—requires that we persist in prayer and stand firm in the Lord as did Daniel, the widow before the judge, and blind Bartemaeus in Mark:

> And they came to Jericho: and as he went out of Jericho with his disciples and a great number of people, blind Bartimaeus, the son of Timaeus, sat by the highway side begging. And when he heard that it was Jesus of Nazareth, he began to cry out, and say, Jesus, thou son of David, have mercy on me. And many charged him that he

should hold his peace: but he cried the more a great deal,
Thou son of David, have mercy on me. And Jesus stood
still, and commanded him to be called. And they call the
blind man, saying unto him, Be of good comfort, rise; he
calleth thee. And he, casting away his garment, rose, and
came to Jesus. And Jesus answered and said unto him,
What wilt thou that I should do unto thee? The blind man
said unto him, Lord, that I might receive my sight. And
Jesus said unto him, Go thy way; thy faith hath made thee
whole. And immediately he received his sight, and followed Jesus in the way.

—MARK 10:46–52

If you have revelation from God's Spirit concerning your
Bible cure, are you willing to persist, standing firm on His
promise of healing to you? We are commanded:

Finally, my brethren, be strong in the Lord, and in the
power of his might. Put on the whole armour of God,
that ye may be able to stand against the wiles of the devil.
For we wrestle not against flesh and blood, but against
principalities, against powers, against the rulers of the
darkness of this world, against spiritual wickedness in
high places. Wherefore take unto you the whole armour
of God, that ye may be able to withstand in the evil day,
and having done all, to stand.

—EPHESIANS 6:10–13

Remember, God does not delay in healing you. In fact, your
healing was purchased on the cross two thousand years ago.
His shed blood has healed you. Isaiah prophetically revealed:
"But he [the Messiah, Jesus] was wounded for our transgres-
sions, he was bruised for our iniquities: the chastisement of
our peace was upon him; and with his stripes we are healed"
(Isa. 53:5; cf. 1 Pet. 2:24). So when we pray for our Bible cure,
we are praying for the manifestation of God's healing that has
already occurred on the cross through the shed blood of Jesus
Christ. In His love, the Father reveals to us our pathway of

healing through His ultimate Bible cure—the shed blood of Jesus Christ.

## Principle #6—Maintain a Violent Attitude Against the Works of Darkness

IN ORDER TO continue in our persistence and standing firm, we must maintain a particular attitude. The greatest danger at this point is that a patient will become passive, give up, or fail to fight this battle. We must be feisty—even violent—in our persistence. "And from the days of John the Baptist until now the kingdom of heaven suffereth violence, and the violent take it by force" (Matt. 11:12).

As Christians, we are called upon to take a unique and unusual action in this verse. Our usual manner in living the Christian life is bearing the fruit of the Spirit with all humility: "But the fruit of the Spirit is love, joy, peace, longsuffering, gentleness, goodness, faith, meekness, temperance: against such there is no law. And they that are Christ's have crucified the flesh with the affections and lusts. If we live in the Spirit, let us also walk in the Spirit" (Gal. 5:22–25).

We manifest these character traits, which are Christ's nature in us, to our fellow man. But toward the devil's wiles and schemes, we manifest violence. When we deal with the works of the devil and the principalities and powers of darkness, we must have an attitude of violence and rise up against the darkness.

How do we become violent toward the kingdom of darkness? Remember that the kingdom of heaven was originally on this earth. Both Adam and Eve enjoyed perfect health—no disease, sickness, illness, or affliction. But now because of sin and our fallen nature, the devil has stolen what should be ours. We must violently take it back. So we declare by faith in the name and authority of Jesus Christ: *No, devil! In Jesus' name, I refuse to accept this disease in my body. In Jesus' name, I command this affliction to flee. My body is the temple of the Holy Spirit. I will not tolerate this attack of the enemy against my body. Disease has no right or authority to exist in my body, the temple of the Holy Spirit, because I have been healed by the stripes, by the shed blood of Jesus Christ. In Jesus' name, I rebuke this sickness.*

Such a violent attitude is necessary to oppose the forces of darkness, putting on the whole armor of God—which is putting on Jesus Himself—and having done all to stand firm! Be feisty and fight back.

Look at the attitude of the four lepers in 2 Kings 7:3–5:

> And there were four leprous men at the entering in of the gate: and they said one to another, Why sit we here until we die? If we say, We will enter into the city, then the famine is in the city, and we shall die there: and if we sit still here, we die also. Now therefore come, and let us fall unto the host of the Syrians: if they save us alive, we shall live; and if they kill us, we shall but die. And they rose up in the twilight, to go unto the camp of the Syrians: and when they were come to the uttermost part of the camp of Syria, behold, there was no man there.

To the person who has done all, I encourage them to have this feisty, even violent, attitude. Don't sit around waiting to die. If God has more for you to do in this life in serving and glorifying Him, then go for it. Having done all, stand firm in your Bible cure and attack the kingdom of darkness with a violent attitude. Let's summarize these principles one more time:

1. *Cast your cares on the Lord* (1 Pet. 5:7).

2. *Pray and petition God for your pathway of healing* (Phil. 4:6–7).

3. *Test your options by the Spirit of God* (Acts 14:27; 6:16; Col. 3:15).

4. *Speak to your mountain* (Mark 11:23–24).

5. *Persist and stand firm in your Bible cure* (Dan. 10; Mark 10:46–53; Luke 18:1–8).

6. *Maintain a violent attitude against the works of darkness* (Matt. 11:12).

God's pathway of healing is set before each of us as we live the Christian life. Through the blood of Jesus Christ, God's Bible cure is available to everyone who trusts in Jesus as Lord and Savior.

# 4

# Records of
# Healings Through the
# Bible Cure

I HAVE BEEN ABLE to watch many of my patients reach total healing from their diseases as they learned to live by the principles that reveal God's pathway of healing. As they learned to identify His specific plan for them and learned to speak to their mountains of disease and command them to fall in submission to the plan of God, they have found the healing for which they were so desperately seeking.

Perhaps you are desperately seeking God's pathway of healing for your own life. I encourage you to keep seeking—God has a pathway just for you. Let the stories in this chapter bring you fresh hope as you read how ten individuals learned to use God's principles to overcome the attack of the enemy against their physical bodies. They were victorious, and today they are finishing the course with joy. YOU CAN, TOO!

## A BIBLE CURE FOR DIABETES

MRS. B., A STRONG Christian lady, came into the clinic after having been diagnosed approximately two years earlier with diabetes. She had been told by her physician that she would need to be on medication, probably for the rest of her life, and she accepted this diagnosis. But being a strong Christian, she began standing on her faith and her belief in God as her Healer. She attended various healing services, and at one healing service she believed that God revealed to her that she had been healed of the diabetes. After being prayed for in the prayer line, she discontinued her diabetes medication. After a few weeks she began feeling very weak in her body. Eventually she returned to her physician, who promptly admitted her to the hospital and started her on insulin.

At this point her future looked bleak. Not only was her diabetes worse than ever, but she was now having symptoms in her body of peripheral neuropathy with numbness and tingling in her legs and lower extremities. In addition, her faith in God had been severely shaken because of her experience in that healing service.

As she entered our clinic, indeed, her situation looked very dismal in the natural. She had severe symptoms in her body, she was discouraged, without hope, and her faith was greatly diminished. Was there indeed a Bible cure for her problem? Was there a pathway for her healing?

After examining this patient, God gave us specific instructions to share with her. She was instructed with very specific things to do in regard to her body. A program of supplements, including high doses of antioxidants to protect the arteries and other organs in her body, was initiated. In addition, she was given higher dosages of B vitamins because of the neuropathy, and she was instructed to begin taking 1,000 micrograms of chromium daily. These substances were all natural substances derived from food and other sources, but higher, more concentrated dosages were needed in her case. She was further instructed in weight loss and given an eating plan for what is considered by many to be the most ideal diet available today—the Mediterranean Diet.

In order to give her hope, we then took her to God's Word, explaining the difference between the healing in Mark, chapter 10; that of blind Bartimaeus, who was healed super-naturally by the word of Jesus and by his faith; and that of the blind man in John, chapter 9, where the anointing of Jesus flowed through a natural substance (mud and saliva). This man's healing came as the result of a process (as he went *his way* to the pool at Saloam). We pointed out to this lady that she too would be healed, in fact, that she *was* healed two thousand years ago by the blood of Jesus. What we were really praying for now was the full manifestation of that healing in her body. We explained that some people are healed in prayer lines supernaturally through their faith and by the laying on of hands; but in other cases, the healing is a process and flows through natural substances as a person follows the instructions of God in obedience. We encouraged her to follow the principles of speaking to her mountain, persisting and standing firm in the Bible cure, and maintaining a violent attitude against the works of darkness (see chapter three for the six principles for healing). We also put her back on a dosage of oral diabetes medication.

It was several months after I had given this lady specific instructions under the leading of the Holy Spirit that she came back to the clinic. Her blood-sugar level was now normal. We did an additional blood test known as a *hemoglobin A1C*, which gives an average blood-sugar level over the last several weeks, and this was also normal. She had lost a significant amount of weight, and we, at this point, cut her oral diabetes medication in half.

In obedience, she continued to follow the program, having a renewed hope in the healing power of Jesus. After three more months, she returned to the clinic and her blood-sugar level was even lower—as was the hemoglobin A1C blood test. She was then told to discontinue the prescription medication and to continue with the other natural substances. Her healing was now manifest. The numbness from the nerve damage in her legs had almost entirely disappeared. Not only did she have a renewed physical body, she had a renewed faith in God as her Healer, simply having understood that the cure for her disease was based on a *process* as healing anointing flowed through the various natural steps to healing that she took.

## A Bible Cure for Heart Disease

Mr. S., a middle-aged gentleman from out of state, journeyed to our clinic in Houston with a most intriguing story. He had progressively developed chest tightness and pressure, even with mild exertion. He consulted with a local family doctor who referred him to a cardiologist. The cardiologist performed various tests, found that three of his coronary arteries were blocked, and advised immediate surgery. This gentleman was a strong Christian, as was his wife, and as they began praying they did not feel at peace about proceeding with surgery. They sought the opinion of another cardiologist. The second cardiologist, after reviewing the prior tests and performing additional tests, concurred with the diagnosis. Again, it was strongly suggested to the patient that if he did not undergo bypass surgery, he would probably not live another year.

Once again, neither the patient nor his wife felt peace about this—but they also did not feel at peace about just ignoring the situation. In their spirits they were sensing that there was something else they needed to do, but they were uncertain about which way to turn.

They had heard about our work with heart patients and about our success with reversing heart disease and artery blockage, so they presented our clinic with a one-inch-thick file containing the records of various procedures including cardiac catheterizations, nuclear studies, echocardiograms, and various other sophisticated medical tests.

I sat down with this patient and his wife and reviewed all the prior data, reviewing carefully the recommendations of the previous cardiologists. Considering traditional medical training, the dictates of current medical practice would indeed tell us to send this man to a cardiovascular surgeon for a triple vessel bypass performed in open-heart surgery.

On the other hand, I did not feel a peace in my spirit about surgery. In many other similar cases with almost the identical data, I have, in fact, been led to recommend surgery for patients, and they, in fact, have done very well. In other cases, however, even with the same medical information and data, the course of healing is different. We were now at a crossroad with this gentleman. He felt no peace about pursuing surgery, yet everything in his chart and everything that modern medicine had taught us dictated that he be admitted immediately for the bypass to increase blood flow to the heart muscle before damage occurred. It was time to follow the principle of testing all his options by the Spirit of God.

After reviewing all the test results, I went into my office, closed the door, and prayed, petitioning God for His specific pathway of healing for this patient. I felt a strong move of the Holy Spirit, revealing that this man was to follow a specified treatment regimen and was not to have surgery. I then called the man and his wife into my office and shared this with them; tears ran down their cheeks as God had spoken the same thing to them.

In cases like this, we can, of course, never know why the Holy Spirit, the One who "will guide you into all truth . . . and . . . shew you things to come" (John 16:13), chooses to guide in a particular direction. However, we do know that things can go wrong during open-heart surgery, and patients can suffer dire complications and consequences of the surgery. Perhaps this man would never have survived open-heart surgery, and only through the leading of the Holy Spirit would we be diverted from this situation.

God outlined a unique program for us to pursue with this gentleman. He was placed on specific vitamins: Vitamin E to help in preventing fat build-up in the arteries; garlic to prevent blood clots from forming on the blockages; low-dose aspirin (derived from the bark of the willow tree), which keeps platelets from clumping together and forming a clot on the roughened areas of the arteries; and other substances such as Co Q-10, which is found in various cereals such as wheat bran and can strengthen the heart contractions. He was also given a specific program of exercise and prescribed a low-dose medicine to dilate the arteries.

This plan was initiated by the Holy Spirit approximately five years ago, and the patient's chest pain is totally gone. He exercises regularly, and he is active in his church and in missionary activity. There was a process of healing for this gentleman involving the use of natural substances, and "as he went his way, he was healed."

## A BIBLE CURE FOR OVARIAN CANCER

MRS. K. WAS diagnosed with ovarian cancer. Ovarian cancer is a very deadly cancer and very difficult to treat and control in the natural. By the time the ovarian cancer was diagnosed, it had already spread to other organs in the abdominal cavity. This lady's diagnosis looked bleak, and she was desperate to find God's pathway for her healing. She was a strong Christian and believed in the power of God to heal. She had prayed about this situation extensively and had others praying for her in the prayer of agreement. The ultimate pathway that led to her healing was a most unusual one.

Under the leading of the Holy Spirit, the clear instruction was given to undergo chemotherapy. She resisted this with her natural mind, but after praying about it, she submitted to the chemotherapy under the direction of a well-known oncologist in Houston who specialized in this type of treatment. A most peculiar turn of events, however, took place. She was scheduled to have a long course of treatment over several weeks—a treatment plan that we knew the Holy Spirit had instructed us to schedule and to begin. However, at the end of only three treatments, the Holy Spirit again spoke with the clear instruction to stop the chemotherapy.

Obviously, this caused a great turmoil at the cancer treatment center. The doctor was furious! The nurses were furious. They were being challenged in their own minds concerning their treatment plans. Yet it was obvious that God had given a different instruction. The lady withdrew from the cancer center clinic and discontinued the chemotherapy. Under our supervision, she began a program of building up her immune system. Ultimately, cancer is a failure of the body's immune system. God designed an active immune system able to recognize abnormal cells and rid the body of them (see chapter six: "Practical Steps You Can Take").

It has now been nine years since the diagnosis of her cancer and her initial treatment. She is entirely cancer-free and without symptoms in her body. The question arises: "Why would God lead her to do only three chemotherapy treatments and then stop the treatment?" Some people even questioned whether we had missed God by doing the chemotherapy in the first place.

I prayed very carefully about this case because of its uniqueness, and God revealed to me precisely why the instructions were given as they were. Chemotherapy is really a poison, and it acts as a double-edged sword. The chemicals in chemotherapy can indeed kill off cancer cells, but at the same time they can weaken the immune system and kill off normal white blood cells in the body. In the unique plan of God, this lady underwent a specified and limited number of chemotherapy treatments to kill out a large number of the cancer cells. However, she did not go through enough of the therapy to depress her own immune system or cause side effects such as hair loss, nausea, and the other common side effects of chemotherapy.

At the end of the three treatments, God's instructions were to begin enhancing her immune system function, and this was done through the use of natural substances. What had actually happened with Mrs. K. was that her immune system had been overwhelmed by the cancer when she began treatment. Once a large number of the cancer cells were killed, then the immune system was strengthened to the point that it overcame the remaining abnormal cells in her body. It was indeed God's specific instruction to start the chemotherapy, proceed with it for only three treatments, and then stop it completely.

Mrs. K. is totally healed today. She is serving God and striving to "finish the course with joy" that God called her to run.

## A Bible Cure for Breast Cancer

Mrs. G. had been diagnosed three years earlier with breast

cancer. She had undergone a limited surgical procedure known as a lumpectomy, in which the cancerous mass was removed, but the breast was not totally removed. However, after a series of tests, it was evident that even though the lumpectomy was done, the "margins were positive." This meant that after the large mass of cancer was removed, there were still cells around the edge of the mass that could continue to grow in her breast. Since the doctors had been unable to get all of the cells with the lumpectomy, the surgeons were now strongly recommending that a radical mastectomy take place, followed by chemotherapy.

Mrs. G. felt no peace about this, and she came to Houston to go through our clinic. After reviewing the medical information, her case did appear, once again, in the natural to be a desperate one.

Cancerous cells left in the body can continue to divide and metastasize and, eventually, lead to death. In talking with Mrs. G., and in conducting her examination, I did not feel it was God's pathway for her to have further surgery, chemotherapy, or any other traditional treatment. She felt the same way as we prayed together and set ourselves in agreement according to the third principle for finding a specific pathway of healing.

In this case, God's instruction was to enhance her own body's immune system and strengthen the cells in her body to fight off the abnormal cancer cells. We set ourselves in agreement in prayer and, at the same time, followed God's specific instruction concerning the nutrition and supplements she was to take. We put her on the food plan that uses foods containing chemicals that fight cancer, as well as other supplements to strengthen the immune system.

Recently, I saw the patient again and, after three years on this treatment and following the above recommendations, her examination was entirely normal. Her mammogram was entirely normal, and there was absolutely no evidence of any cancer in her body. She knew in her spirit, as I did, that she was cancer-free. Mrs. G. was spared the trauma of a radical mastectomy and chemotherapy as she followed God's specific plan of healing for her body.

## A BIBLE CURE FOR A
## MISDIAGNOSED HEART CONDITION

PASTOR M. REPORTED to me that he would notice a strange sensation in his chest area prior to preaching, which he described as a mild pressure or flutter in the chest area. He consulted with a physician and was referred to a cardiologist. The cardiologist detected a spasm occurring in the coronary artery, and the pastor was put on several medications and told to limit his activity. His insurance company refused to issue him insurance because of the findings of this test.

He did not feel right about this diagnosis. He underwent an examination. Pastor M. was a vigorous man, full of God, and I knew something was just not right about his diagnosis. I tested him, performing several heart-related tests including a maximal treadmill stress test, which was perfectly normal. I then reviewed all of his prior medical studies, which included two previous heart catheterizations.

In this case the diagnosis was wrong. There was a slight spasm in one of the arteries, but it was caused by the tip of the catheter that was used to inject dye into the heart. There was no blockage in any artery whatsoever. In fact, a second catheterization revealed no evidence of spasm or artery blockage or other problems with the heart. The enemy tried to use this diagnosis to bring despair, but God's truth prevailed. The original symptoms (flutter and chest pressure) were simply muscular in nature.

He was an active exerciser, but during the course of testing he was found to have very high cholesterol levels. God then gave us additional instruction. The good news was that his heart was strong and his arteries were all normal. But because of the high cholesterol, he did, in fact, face future heart disease and blockage in the arteries. In this case, God used the misdiagnosis to alert us to a problem that would occur years in the future. So we then initiated treatment that would bring the blood levels down.

In this case, a chemical that was derived from a plant known as aspergillus was used. This plant-derived pill is taken once daily, and studies show that this medicine can reduce the risk of heart disease and stroke 40 to 50 percent. The pastor received good news on two counts: One—he did not have any problem with his heart. Two—out of obedience to God, he would be spared from any future heart problems because of the recognition of the cholesterol problem and God's provision and pathway to get the cholesterol level down.

## A BIBLE CURE FOR NERVES AND MUSCLES

MRS. T., THE next case study, is a lady who had been to six different physicians complaining of multiple symptoms in her body. She described joint pain, recurring problems with fatigue, and tenderness in various muscle groups. In fact, she was really feeling so bad that she could hardly function. The doctors performed multiple tests—thousands of dollars' worth—and had been unable to diagnose the problem. Some thought she had lupus. Some thought she had rheumatoid arthritis, and some thought she needed to be admitted to the psychiatric unit.

She came into the clinic believing that God had a pathway for her healing, but she was desperate to find an answer. I began questioning this lady, and I discovered that her symptoms began rather suddenly after a case of the flu approximately two years earlier. She got over the flu all right, but she was left with the symptoms of muscle tenderness, aching, and fatigue that had progressively worsened. Her life was in shambles, and her husband was at his wit's end. They had prayed together. They had been in prayer lines. Their pastor had counseled them, but her healing eluded her.

I questioned her very carefully about the beginning of her symptoms, and she was certain that they began after a specific infection. She could even remember the month and year that the flu had occurred. We began examining her body and at the same time began praying and seeking the leading of the Holy Spirit to guide us to truth about her diagnosis and treatment.

The diagnosis quickly became obvious. She had fibromyalgia. This is a disease that is a close cousin of the chronic fatigue syndrome in which various muscle groups become very tender to touch. Patients with this think they have arthritis, rheumatism, and various ailments. What actually happens with this disease, we believe, is that there is an overreaction or overactivity of the immune system, often following an infection or a stressful event in one's life. This is why the Holy Spirit led me to question her about the infection. What frequently occurs is that there is an overreaction of the immune system, and the immune system eliminates the virus or the bacteria from the body but then stays activated. This causes the symptoms of tenderness in the muscles…and the fatigue. It can even affect brain chemicals and lead to depression.

A fresh hope began to emerge as Mrs. T. began to understand the nature of her problem. The Bible tells us that we should not be unaware of the schemes or devices of the enemy. (See Luke 21:34.) Once we understand the schemes and devices of the enemy, we can apply Mark 11:23 by speaking specifically to the "mountain," which in her case was actually an overactive immune system.

God then gave us a specific way to pray, and He showed us how His anointing was to rest on certain natural substances that would bring her immune system back into proper balance. I saw this lady several weeks after the initial visit, and her symptoms were totally gone. She, in fact, almost appeared to be a different person, with a renewed faith in her God and a renewed vigor in her physical body.

## A BIBLE CURE FOR DEPRESSION

MRS. W. CAME into the clinic after being diagnosed by two other physicians with depression. She had experienced severe mood changes, and it seemed almost as if her entire personality had changed. She was a strong Christian with a sweet personality, but for a period of approximately twelve months, these changes had turned her into an angry, suspicious, and withdrawing person. Her personality changes were putting a tremendous strain on a previously strong marriage. Her husband even called me on the phone prior to her visit and said, "Something is going to have to be done, or we may not be able to stay together much longer."

How is the Bible cure going to intervene in this situation? We examined this lady, and it was evident quickly, through the revelation of the Holy Spirit, that although she had suffered mood changes, they were not caused by depression. They were caused by changes related to a hormonal imbalance. She was only in her mid-forties, and other doctors had not considered a hormonal problem because of her age. But tests revealed that she was very deficient in estrogen. God led us to use a plant-derived, natural-type estrogen with her.

Within eight weeks she was a different person. She was once again a loving wife and a caring Christian; the changes in her body were simply the result of hormonal changes. God placed various estrogens in plants, for instance, known as phytoestrogens that can prevent and reverse the symptoms of estrogen deficiency but will not increase the risk of breast and other cancers. Missed diagnoses are often one of Satan's most vicious tricks to keep God's people under bondage and discouragement and to keep them from finishing with joy the course to which God has called them.

## A BIBLE CURE FOR ARTHRITIS

MRS. D. WAS in her mid-sixties and suffering severe problems with her knee. She had been to two orthopedic surgeons, and both of them had recommended that she have knee replacement surgery. It was getting to the point that she could hardly walk. She was desperate for a solution to this problem, but she simply did not feel good about surgery.

We examined her and conducted various tests on her, ruling out rheumatic disease and other problems in her body that might cause the knee problem. Her diagnosis was osteoarthritic changes at the knee joint, induced by cartilage thinning. This is commonly known as "the wear-and-tear form" of arthritis. We placed her on a regimen of 1,500 milligrams of glucosamine daily in divided dosages and 1,200 milligrams of chondroitin sulfate daily in divided dosages.

We continued this program for several months before she returned to the clinic. When she did, there was a big smile on her face, and it was obvious to me that she was walking very differently than when I first saw her. Indeed, the cartilage had been repaired to a significant extent, surgery was no longer a consideration, and she was now able to carry on with her normal daily activities.

## A BIBLE CURE FOR STOMACH CANCER

MRS. P., A sweet lady in her sixties who was a pastor's wife, had been diagnosed several weeks earlier with stomach cancer. She was progressively losing weight and getting weaker and weaker. She and her husband came to the clinic together, and I examined her and talked with her extensively. We had to have a word from God, as her condition was deteriorating rapidly. I completed all of her tests, and I was puzzled because I knew there was something we were missing. I had the strong impression that God wanted to heal this lady, but I sensed there was a hindrance that was interfering with the manifestation of healing.

We had finished the testing when God suddenly spoke to me, revealing the reason Mrs. P. could not get healed. This was a very interesting situation because this lady was one of the sweetest, kindest Christian women you could ever meet. She simply glowed with the gentleness of Jesus. God clearly spoke to me and revealed that she was not able to get her healing because she was too meek and gentle concerning this foreign invader in her body. God quickened me to send for her husband, who was a sweet man of God, and he came into my office. I asked the pastor to sit down and began to share the fact that I knew why his wife could not get her healing.

As I began sharing what God had revealed about Mrs. P.'s illness with her husband, the tears ran down his cheeks, and he nodded his head in agreement. He already knew what I was telling him. I told him that the Holy Spirit revealed that she could not get her healing because she could not rise up with a feisty, fighting attitude and resist this work of darkness in her body. I reminded him of Matthew 11:12, where it says: "The kingdom of heaven suffereth violence, and the violent take it by force."

Mrs. P.'s basic problem was that she was very passive and accepting of this disease in her body. She simply could not rise up, resist it, speak to it, and command it with authority to leave her body. Her husband told me that he had been trying for months and months to arouse the same attitude in her spirit, but that she simply would not do it.

A few months later, I heard from him that she had gone on home to be with the Lord. Many secular studies are currently showing that indeed those with a feisty, fighting attitude are often the ones that overcome cancer and other diseases. It is the patients who do not passively accept treatment, but who vigorously fight off the disease and literally do battle with it that succeed more than those who passively accept the disease as their so-called fate in life.

## A BIBLE CURE FOR THE IMMUNE SYSTEM

THE NEXT CASE study, Mrs. A., is a lady with multiple allergies. She had suffered greatly and gone to many doctors, but none of them were able to help her. (Her story reminds me of the woman with the issue of blood in Mark 5, who suffered at the hands of many physicians.) Mrs. A. stated that she had taken every kind of antihistamine and decongestant available, even traveling to a world-renowned allergy clinic where she was placed on multiple medications, but nothing seemed to work. She began losing her strength and became nauseated; she was desperately seeking God for a way out. Though her life was not in danger, she was unable to function on a day-to-day basis because the symptoms in her body were so severe. Did God have a Bible cure for her?

When she came into the clinic, we evaluated her in our usual manner. Our approach is to evaluate every major system in the body. Often medicine focuses on one organ or one area (the one that the patient is complaining about), but in reality, a problem in one part of the body may be caused by an abnormality somewhere else. Therefore, we do not focus on one area, but we do a complete head-to-toe evaluation, looking at the body as a whole.

Having completed these tests and after praying with this woman, God clearly outlined her pathway to healing. We needed first to apply Mark 11:23 to her situation by instructing her specifically as to what her "mountain" was. If she was to speak to her mountain, she had to have a clear understanding as to what the specific attack of the enemy was. We explained that the allergy symptoms were due to an excessively sensitive and overly reactive immune system, which was recognizing harmless substances such as dust pollen and mold as being harmful, thus secreting various substances to try to neutralize and eliminate these things from her body. We further explained that she needed to speak to her immune system and command it to come into balance and to stop recognizing harmless things as being harmful to her.

On the natural side, we prescribed a program to balance the immune system. The immune system is really God's natural hedge against external factors that can harm the body. If the immune system, however, becomes overactive, it can cause allergies, turning to attack the body itself, causing autoimmune diseases such as lupus and rheumatoid arthritis. God has given us various chemicals within foods and plants that can balance the immune system. According to Proverbs 18:9, we began finding what endeavors this lady needed to do herself to bring about her healing:

> He who is loose and slack in his work is brother to him who is a destroyer [and he who does not use his endeavors to heal himself is brother to him who commits suicide].
>
> —AMP

As she began praying in the specific way God instructed, and as she balanced her immune system according to the directions we had been given by the Holy Spirit, her symptoms totally disappeared, and she once again resumed a normal lifestyle. Once again the Bible cure proved to be the answer when all of the sophisticated allergy testing and allergy medication had failed (see "Balancing the Immune System," chapter six).

These stories are just a few of the victorious healings I have seen take place as individuals begin to walk upon the specific paths of healing God had ordained as the answers to their medical conditions and diseases. We share these principles of healing daily in our medical practice. I am awed continually by the awesome healing power of God.

Yes, we would all like to be healed instantly, supernaturally, and miraculously. Thank God that miracles are still taking place. Jesus is the "same yesterday, today and forever" (Heb. 13:8). Seek God for the specific pathway that will lead to your healing. Apply the principles you are learning in this book to your life, and find a doctor who understands these principles also and will pray in agreement with you.

No matter what your problem or illness, God has a pathway for that manifestation of healing to take place. Let your hope soar and your faith increase as you wait expectantly to realize your healing.

# 5

# Healthy Eating With the Mediterranean Diet

A GREAT INTEREST HAS arisen in medical and health circles today about the foods that have been eaten for centuries in the lands of the Bible. The diet of Middle Eastern people is of particular interest.

One name given to this group of foods that prevent disease and help to cure diseases is the "Mediterranean Diet." This diet is very similar to the one described in Genesis.

> אשר על־פני כל־הארץ ואת־כל־העץ אשר־בו פרי־עץ זרע זרע לכם
> ויאמר אלהים הנה נתתי לכם את־כל־עשב זרע זרע. And God said,
> Behold, I have given you every herb bearing seed, which
> is upon the face of all the earth, and every tree, in the
> which is the fruit of a tree yielding seed; to you it shall be
> for meat.
>
> —GENESIS 1:29

> אשר הוא־הי לכם יהיה לאכלה כירק עשב נתתי לכם את־כל . . .
> כל־רמש. Every moving thing that liveth shall be meat for

you; even as the green herb have I given you all things.
—GENESIS 9:3

We will identify some of the specific foods mentioned in the Bible cure throughout the Old and New Covenants, and then observe the foods that are eaten today in those same regions around the Mediterranean Sea. I will list the specific foods mentioned in the Bible cure and then describe more generally the food groups you should eat in order to enjoy the health benefits that are rooted in the Bible cure's Mediterranean Diet.

## SPECIFIC FOODS MENTIONED IN THE BIBLE CURE

THE BIBLE CURE gives us specific commands about two things: First we are to avoid certain fats: "It shall be a perpetual statute for your generations . . . that ye eat neither fat nor blood" (Lev. 3:17). Second, we are to avoid obesity: "And take heed to yourselves, lest at any time your hearts be over-charged with surfeiting, and drunkenness, and cares of this life, and so that day come upon you unawares. For as a snare shall it come on all them that dwell on the face of the whole earth" (Luke 21:34–35).

In addition to the foods we are to avoid eating, the Bible cure mentions the following specific foods, which are found throughout the Mediterranean Diet and should be the source of food for us today.

- Clean, lean meat from animals with divided hooves; animals that are cud-chewing (Lev. 11:2–3)

- Fish with fins *and* scales (Lev. 11:9; Deut. 14:9)

- Cucumbers, melons, leeks, onions, and garlic (Num. 11:5)

- Grapes and wine (Deut. 8:7–9; John 15)

- Wheat, barley, vines (grapes), figs, pomegranates, olive oil, and honey (Deut. 8:8)

- Raisins and apples (Song of Sol. 2:5, AMP)

- Bread (Exod. 12:8, 15; Ezek. 4:9)

- Beans (Ezek. 4:9)

- Honey, pistachio nuts, and almonds (Gen. 43:11, AMP)

- Yogurt and the milk of cows, sheep, and goats (Isa. 7:15, 22; Prov. 27:27, AMP)

## Foods in Old Testament Times

א Like many Arabs today, the Hebrews ate meat only on festive occasions. To vary the monotonous daily diet of parched or cooked wheat and barley, the Hebrew housewife would grind the grain into coarse flour, mix it with olive oil, and bake it into flat cakes of bread. She garnished the cakes with lentils, broad beans, and other vegetables. Cucumbers, onions, leeks, and garlic perked up bland dishes. Fresh and dried fruit and wild honey sweetened the meals. In a water-short land, the Hebrews heartily quaffed wine and prized the milk of goats and sheep.

Solomon and his sumptuous court demanded richer fare for their golden table. "Solomon's daily provisions were thirty cors of fine flour [about 335 bushels] and sixty cors of meal, ten head of stall-fed cattle, twenty of pasture-fed cattle and a hundred sheep and goats, as well as deer, gazelles, roebucks and choice fowl" (1 Kings 4:22–23, NIV).

We can even get a glimpse into the everyday life of Mary, Joseph, and Jesus, and we find that their dinner table held many of the same foods as those provided by Solomon to his people:

In her daily rounds [the Jewish maiden Mary] she would have fetched water, tended the fire, and ground grain. The family dined on a porridge of wheat or barley groats, supplemented by beans, lentils, cucumbers, and other vegetables—with onions, leeks, garlic, and olive oil for seasoning. For dessert came dates, figs, and pomegranates. Watered wine was the universal drink. Only on feast days did humble Galileans eat meat.[1]

## THE MEDITERRANEAN DIET

*THE BIBLE CURE* identifies some of the basic foods found in the Mediterranean Diet, which offers a healthy basis for eating that is rooted in the truths of the ancient Hebrew texts. Let's examine some of the specific foods eaten by those in the ancient world to see how they help us to prevent and cure disease.

There has been a great interest developing in what is known as the "Mediterranean Diet." This diet is very similar to one outlined in Genesis 1:29 and Genesis 9:3. It seems that the diet followed by people living along the Mediterranean Sea results in some of the lowest rates of colon cancer, breast cancer, and coronary heart disease in the world. Why would this be?

It is no accident that Israel is one of these Mediterranean countries. I believe that most of this diet can be traced back to the Bible cure guidelines given to God's chosen people—the Israelites.

Mediterranean countries have developed their own dishes, but these dishes share several characteristics. As you take a look at the ingredients used in these menus, you will observe that the following foods are consumed daily:

1. *Olive oil.* Olive oil replaces most fats, oils, butter, and margarine; it is used in salads as well as for cooking. Olive oil raises levels of the good cholesterol (HDL) and may strengthen immune system function. Extra-virgin olive oil is the preferred one to use.

2. *Breads.* Bread is consumed daily and is prepared as dark, chewy, crusty loaves. The typical American sliced white bread and wheat breads are not used in the Mediterranean countries.

3. *Pasta, rice, couscous, bulgur, potatoes.* Pasta is often served with fresh vegetables and herbs

sautéed in olive oil; occasionally it is served with small quantities of lean beef. Dark rice is preferred. Couscous and bulgur are other forms of wheat.

4. *Grains*. The Mediterranean Diet includes many sources of grains. To obtain the same healthy grains, eat cereals containing wheat bran (one-half cup, four to five times weekly); alternate with a cereal such as Bran Buds (one-half cup) or those that contain oat bran (one-third cup).

5. *Fruits*. The Mediterranean Diet includes many fruits, preferably raw. Eat two to three pieces daily.

6. *Beans*. It includes many kinds of beans, including pintos, great northern, navy, and kidney beans. Bean and lentil soups are very popular (prepared with a small amount of olive oil). We should have at least one-half cup of beans, three to four times weekly.

7. *Nuts*. Almonds (ten per day) or walnuts (ten per day) rank at the top of the list of acceptable nuts in the Mediterranean Diet.

8. *Vegetables*. Dark green vegetables are prominent, especially in salads. To obtain the same benefits in our diet, we should eat at least one of the following vegetables daily: cabbage, broccoli, cauliflower, turnip greens, or mustard greens; and one of the following groups of vegetables daily: carrots, spinach, sweet potatoes, cantaloupe, peaches, or apricots.

9. *Cheese and yogurt*. Unlike milk and milk products, some recent studies indicate that cheese may not contribute as much to clogged arteries as was previously believed. In the Mediterranean Diet, cheese

may be grated on soups or a small wedge may be combined with a piece of fruit for dessert; use the reduced-fat varieties (the fat-free often taste like rubber). The best yogurt is fat-free, but not frozen.

In addition to these healthy foods that are included in the Mediterranean Diet on a daily basis, there are some foods that should be included in your diet only a few times weekly. These include:

10. *Fish*. The healthiest fish are "cold-water" varieties such as cod, salmon, and mackerel; trout is also good. These fish are high in omega-3 fatty acids.

11. *Poultry*. Poultry can be eaten two to three times weekly; white breast meat from which the skin has been removed is the best.

12. *Eggs*. Eggs should be eaten in small amounts (two to three per week).

13. *Red meat*. Red meat should only be included in your diet on an average of three times a month. Use only lean cuts with the fat trimmed; it can also be used in small amounts as an additive to spice up soup or pasta. The severe restriction of red meat in the Mediterranean Diet is a radical departure from the American diet, but it is a major contributor to the low rates of cancer and heart disease found in these countries.

## EATING THE MEDITERRANEAN WAY

A TYPICAL MEDITERRANEAN breakfast would consist of dark bread or cereal (such as those mentioned above), a piece of fresh fruit, and perhaps a small amount of yogurt or a slice of cheese. Lunch or dinner would very likely include:

1. *Salads.* The salad is eaten with each meal; it is made of fresh greens (and other vegetables) with added olive oil, vinegar, and/or lemon juice.

2. *Soups.* Soups are often made with chopped celery, garlic, carrots, onions, and other vegetables and cooked in a chicken stock or other liquid. They are seasoned with added herbs; a small amount of grated cheese (use low-fat) is sprinkled for garnish on top.

3. *Pasta.* A staple of many meals, fresh pasta is often mixed with fresh vegetables and herbs that have been sautéed in olive oil. Occasionally a bit of beef or chicken is added to the pasta dish.

4. *Rice.* Rice is a prominent addition in this diet. Many different rices are used, including the dark, brown, and wild rices. These are prepared in many creative ways, including rice pilafs, risottos, and thick soups and stews.

5. *Staple items.* Many fruits and vegetables are staples in the Mediterranean Diet. Tomatoes, onions, and peppers are used often. Olive oil is used often in cooking and salads instead of heavy oils.

## THE MEDITERRANEAN FOOD PYRAMID

THE FOOD PYRAMID on the next page summarizes the eating habits of people who eat the Mediterranean way. In the pages following the pyramid, notice the balance between the amounts of each category of food in this diet.

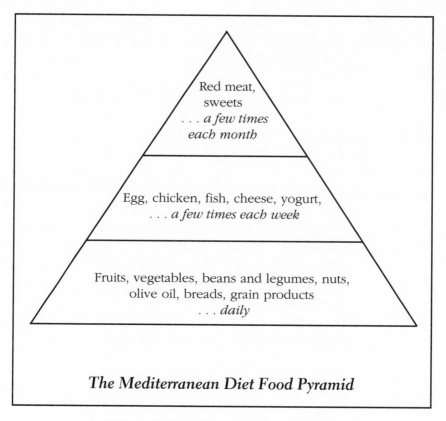

Red meat,
sweets
. . . *a few times
each month*

Egg, chicken, fish, cheese, yogurt,
. . . *a few times each week*

Fruits, vegetables, beans and legumes, nuts,
olive oil, breads, grain products
. . . *daily*

**The Mediterranean Diet Food Pyramid**

## A "NEW WINE" FOR YOUR HEALTH

THERE HAVE BEEN over fifty research articles from universities indicating the health benefits from wine (particularly red wine). Since the Bible talks so much about wine, Linda and I researched the subject and discovered that red wine contains a useful substance (resveratrol). Researchers at the University of Illinois have found that resveratrol inhibits cancer by helping to prevent DNA damage to cells, keeping cells from transforming into cancer, and thus preventing the growth and spread of cancer. Resveratrol has been shown to lower cholesterol in recent Cornell University studies.

Other substances in red wine known as biologically active flavonoids are potent antioxidants. Antioxidants neutralize free radicals, which may be the root cause of cancer, heart disease, cataracts, rheumatoid arthritis, and the aging process itself. Flavonoids can also protect us from strokes and heart attacks by reducing platelet aggregation, which allows the blood to flow more smoothly through the blood vessels.

God, in His infinite wisdom, has now shown us how to get the benefits of wine without the alcohol; Linda and I use a non-alcoholic red wine made by Ariel (a type of wine known as a Cabernet Sauvignon). You will have to search around to find it, or you can call 1-800-456-9472 for information. You should drink six to twelve ounces daily to gain the benefits mentioned above. The thought of drinking "wine" is foreign to many, but, without the alcohol, we can obtain all the benefits God intended without the detriments.

Pray about this; God may use this as a part of your pathway to healing and health.

## God's Nutrition Laws

When the Bible speaks to the issue of the healing of our physical bodies, it illustrates clearly a supernatural aspect and a natural aspect of divine health. In this section, we will deal with the natural, practical things that God wants us do in order to walk in divine health.

In Exodus 23:25, God said that He would "bless thy bread, and thy water; and I will take sickness from the midst of thee." This clearly indicates that the practical aspects of people's nutrition contribute prominently in being free of sickness. Let's take a look at nutrition from a biblical perspective.

In the fifteenth chapter of Exodus, God entered into a healing covenant with man:

> If thou wilt diligently hearken to the voice of the LORD thy God, and wilt do that which is right in his sight, and wilt give ear to his commandments, and keep all his statutes, I will put none of these diseases upon thee, which I have brought upon the Egyptians: for I am the LORD that healeth thee.
>
> —Exodus 15:26

Immediately after establishing this covenant of healing with His people, in the sixteenth chapter of Exodus God addressed the issue of nutrition by providing manna to His people. This supernatural, nutritionally sound substance sustained the Israelites for the forty years that they wandered in the wilderness.

When the Israelites reached the Promised Land, they discovered a land rich in nutrition, filled with all the natural provisions of God to enable them to develop the sound, nutritious meal plan that has today become known as the Mediterranean Diet.

The things we eat have always had a direct bearing on the condition of our health. Six of the ten leading causes of death in this country today deal with the issue of what we eat.

## WHAT SHOULD I BE EATING?

WE HAVE ALREADY looked at some of the foods that are healthy for us. Let's look again, this time considering the essential nutrient compounds for a healthy diet and the foods that provide each nutrient to our body.

### Protein

While protein is essential to our health, we should limit our protein intake to 10 to 15 percent of our total calories. Excessive amounts of protein can lead to kidney problems, high cholesterol levels, and heart disease, as well as other health-related problems.

Limit red meats to three servings monthly. Emphasize fish (especially trout, salmon, cod, and tuna) and chicken (preferably the white meat without the skin).

### Carbohydrates

God set the pattern for our nutritional intake in the Book of Genesis:

And God said, See, I have given you every plant yielding seed that is on the face of all the land, and every tree with seed in its fruit; you shall have them for food.

—Genesis 1:29, AMP

Every moving thing that lives shall be food for you; and as I give you the green vegetables and plants, I give you everything.

—Genesis 9:3, AMP

The verse from the first chapter of Genesis above deals with the natural foods God gave us to meet our nutritive need for carbohydrates. Grains, seeds, fruits, and vegetables are the sources we have available to us for carbohydrates.

Complex carbohydrates are vitally important to our healthy bodies. There are some people groups in the world today (particularly in Asian countries) where hardening of the arteries and cancer are almost nonexistent—due to a diet consisting primarily of complex carbohydrates.

The main focus of your food intake should come from the following groups of complex carbohydrates:

- *Green/yellow vegetables*—three or more servings daily

- *Grains, including cereal, rice, whole-grain breads*—two servings daily

- *Fruits*—three or more daily

- *Beans and peas*—two to three servings weekly

Certain carbohydrate-rich vegetables and fruits show cancer-protective effects. These include:

- *Those high in vitamin A*

These fruits and vegetables are often orange or yellow in color. They include apricots, carrots, cantaloupe, pumpkin, peaches, and sweet potatoes. Other very good complex-carbohydrate sources are watermelon, broccoli, collard greens, romaine lettuce, and tomatoes.

- *Those high in vitamin C*

Vitamin C-rich food sources include cantaloupe, broccoli, collard greens, oranges, cabbage, tomatoes, strawberries, cauliflower, and spinach.

- *Cruciferous vegetables*

Eat at least some of these vegetables several times a week. They include broccoli, cabbage, Brussel sprouts, and cauliflower.

Carbohydrates are mentioned frequently in the Bible. One of the best examples of a high complex-carbohydrate diet in the Bible cure can be seen in the example of Daniel. When Daniel and his friends refused to eat the rich, fat-laden, unhealthy foods from the king's table, Daniel appealed to the king's steward for a different menu:

> Then said Daniel to the steward . . . Prove your servants, I beseech you, for ten days, and let us be given a vegetable diet and water to drink. Then let our appearance and the appearance of the youths who eat of the king's rich dainties be observed and compared by you, and deal with us your servants according to what you see. So [the man] consented to them in this matter and proved them ten days. And at the end of ten days it was seen that they were looking better and had taken on more flesh than all the youths who ate of the king's rich dainties. So the steward took away their rich dainties, and the wine they were to drink, and gave them vegetables.
> —DANIEL 1:11–16, AMP

What a great example Daniel and his friends are to us of the healthy benefits from a carbohydrate-rich diet.

## Fiber

Fiber is essential in your daily diet. There are many sources of fiber, including not only fruits and vegetables, but also many grains. Consider some of the following choices for fiber:

- *Wheat fiber* from bran-type cereals. Wheat fiber has been proven to be successful in preventing certain types of cancer. Try to get one-half cup of bran cereal daily.

- *Oat fiber (oat bran)* may lower blood-fat levels (cholesterol). Consider including one-third cup of an oat bran cereal daily (may be mixed with wheat bran).

- *Beans and peas* should be eaten regularly (preferably three times weekly). Include great northern, pinto, limas, and lentils, all of which seem to lower cholesterol (blood fats).

## Fats

God's harshest words about nutrition concern fats:

> It shall be a perpetual statute for your generations throughout all your dwellings, that ye eat neither fat nor blood.
>
> —LEVITICUS 3:17

Forty-two percent of the American diet is fat. We rank among the highest percentage group of people in the world for heart disease and hardening of the arteries. You will need to give close consideration to your fat intake. You can successfully lower your fat consumption and pave the pathway to better health by following these simple guidelines:

- *Eat lean red meat sparingly.* Emphasize fish and chicken in your diet.

- *Limit cheese.* Cheese is often more than 50 percent fat; eat skim-milk, low-fat, or nonfat cheeses.

- *Oils.* Read labels for "coconut or palm oil" and avoid these products. Watch out for coffee creamers, artificial dairy toppings, and hydrogenated or partially hydrogenated oils.

Certain types of fat can be good to include in your diet. Substitute these good fats for those that are unhealthy for you to eat. They include:

- *Canola oil.* This oil may actually lower blood fat levels; use it for cooking, in recipes, and for salad dressings.

- *Olive oil.* Olive oil is good for you—it may lower blood fats. Some studies suggest that it may also lower blood pressure. Use it on salads, for cooking, as a substitute in many recipes, and in place of margarine.

- *Certain oily fish* such as tuna, salmon, and cod may lower the tendency to develop blood clots and heart disease.

## Sugar

Be careful with simple sugars; limit them in your diet—they are too high in calories. Sugar-laden desserts are often high in saturated fat. At the present time, sugar substitutes seem to be safe. Aspartame is actually a combination of natural amino acids that occurs in peaches, green beans, milk, and in many common substances. Some people, however, tolerate aspartame poorly and should avoid it, as it can occasionally cause headaches, allergies, and other reactions. Although saccharin seems to be safe, aspartame, being natural, is the preferred choice.

## Salt

Salt, or sodium chloride, is necessary to our body, but it can be extremely harmful if overused. Do not add salt when you are cooking, and do not add it at the table on prepared food. If you must "spice up" the taste of your food, consider a salt substitute or a "lite" salt. Be creative with some of the herb-combination substitutes available today. Don't use salt tablets—they have no nutritive value to a healthy diet.

## Coffee

The caffeine in coffee (in excessive amounts) can increase cholesterol levels, cause heart irregularities, and may contribute to discomfort from fibrocystic disease in women. Limit your coffee intake to two cups of regular coffee daily; the rest should be decaffeinated.

## HOW TO SHOP FOR FOOD

WHEN GOD ENTERED a healing covenant with man, He immediately shifted the focus to what His people should eat, giving specific instructions as to how they should gather and prepare their food. (See Exodus 15:26.) In Exodus 23:25 God promised to place a blessing on the bread and water (the daily food) of His people. With His blessing, God indicated that He would "take sickness away from the midst of thee."

The Surgeon General of the United States, in just the past few months, has reaffirmed God's nutritional laws by stating: "Your choice of diet can influence your long-term health prospects more than any other action you might take."

The following section will help you prepare to examine your diet and to determine to choose the foods for you and your family that will bring you the ultimate opportunity for good health. Choose wisely—your health, and that of your family, will be affected by your choices.

## Buying Fresh Produce

* Add more produce to your diet. There are many varieties from which to choose.

- Romaine lettuce is the best choice in the lettuce family.

- Choose produce known to be good sources of vitamin C: peppers, tomatoes, broccoli, cabbage, potatoes, greens (collard, mustard, turnip), cantaloupe, honeydew, kiwi, and strawberries.

- Eat the skins of fruits and vegetables.

- Select produce high in vitamin A: deep colored green, yellow, and orange vegetables; include spaghetti squash, yellow squash, and zucchini.

- Make delicious soups from a wide variety of vegetables.

## Delicatessen Choices

- Select sliced roast beef, turkey, or lean ham that is 97–98 percent fat-free.

- Use bacon sparingly, if at all. When using bacon, use Canadian bacon, which is low in fat (but high in sodium).

- Avoid hot dogs—even those made with turkey and chicken—they are high in fat.

## Selecting Dairy Foods

- Use plain nonfat yogurt as a substitute for sour cream.

- Choose nonfat or low-fat cheeses, or cheese with less than five grams of fat per ounce such as Alpine Lace Swiss cheese, mozzarella, scamorze, ricotta, and nonfat cottage cheese.

- Use fat-free milk.

- Try buttermilk—it's low in fat.

- Use only small amounts of margarine, preferably choosing the new nonfat varieties that have no transfatty acids; extra-virgin olive oil can be used instead of margarine.

## The Array of Breads and Cereals

- Use whole-wheat and whole-grain breads (rye, oat bran, oat nut).

- When selecting cereals, it is best to combine wheat bran and oat bran, choosing brands such as All Bran and Fiber One (eat one-third to one-half cup daily of these type cereals). When selecting a cereal made of oat bran alone, such as Quaker Oat Bran, eat one-third cup daily. Wheat helps to protect the colon; oat lowers cholesterol.

- Be wary of granola-type cereals. Often they contain too much fat.

## Surveying the Meat Counter

- Avoid animal fat as much as possible, as well as organ meats such as liver and sweetbreads.

- Use lean, trimmed cuts of meat—flank steaks, round steaks, sirloins, tenderloins, and ground sirloin, round, and chuck.

- Pork is generally very high in fat; the tenderloin of pork is lowest in fat (26 percent); bacon is one of the highest (80 percent).

- Choose *select* instead of *choice* or *prime* cuts of meat.

- Limit, or avoid, ribs, corned beef, sausage, and bacon.

## Fish and Poultry Choices

- Choose fish from deep, cold-water regions. This includes salmon, tuna, mackerel, sea trout, herring, and cod.

- Limit your intake of shrimp; use lobster and crab sparingly.

- Fresh ground turkey is a good substitute for ground beef.

- Whole turkey or turkey breast steaks are excellent choices of meat.

- When eating chicken, remember that half of the calories in chicken are in the skin—discard the skin before cooking. To keep chicken moist during cooking, baste with olive oil.

## Finding Frozen Foods

- Choose frozen dinners with less than fifteen milligrams fat, less than four hundred calories, and less than eight hundred milligrams of sodium.

- Buy frozen juice concentrates to make juice.

- Use iced milk and nonfat frozen yogurt instead of ice cream.

- Frozen juice bars and frozen fruit bars without added sugar are good dessert choices.

## Choosing Fats, Oils, and Dressings

- Use vegetable oil for cooking—the best choice is extra-virgin olive oil; canola oil is a good second choice.

- Olive oil is the best choice for salads. Or prepare or

purchase one of the wonderful no-oil dressings available now.

- Use low-fat, no cholesterol vegetable spray (such as Pam) instead of oil or butter.

- A butter substitute such as Butterbuds can be used on potatoes and other vegetables, or as a spread for breads and rolls.

- Use fat-free mayonnaise.

- Use diet dressings that contain less than ten calories per tablespoon.

- Use low-fat or fat-free Italian dressings for salads and as a marinade for meat, poultry, and vegetables.

- Use seasoned vinegars, lemon juice, or herb and spice blends on vegetables and fish or chicken.

## Packaged Products

- Avoid palm, palm kernel, and coconut oils (read the labels before you buy).

- Unsalted pretzels are a good low-fat snack.

- Microwave popcorn is often high in fat (the wrong kind of fat) and salt—use air-popped popcorn instead.

- Use potato chips sparingly. When you do purchase chip products, select the no-salt, fat-free choices available now.

- There are several types of dried beans to choose that will lower cholesterol. These include great northern, pinto, kidney, and navy beans.

- Choose rice wisely—long-grained brown rice is a good choice.

- Cookies are usually high in fat (read the labels)—buy cookies only if they contain *no* palm or coconut oil and have no more than three grams of fat per cookie. Try cookies made with fruit juices and no hydrogenated oils (found in the health food section).

## What About Canned Foods?

- Avoid fruit punches and drinks; use 100-percent pure fruit juice.

- Select canned fish with edible bones such as salmon or sardines (watch the sodium levels in canned fish).

- Canned beans, peas, and corn are all good sources of vitamins, minerals, and fiber. However, they are not as nutritious as fresh—use them for convenience only when necessary.

### EZEKIEL BREAD

THE BIBLE CURE actually recommends a particular bread to eat. Since it is described in Ezekiel, I have called it *Ezekiel Bread.*

> Also take wheat, barley, beans, lentils, millet and spelt, and put them into one vessel and make bread of them…
> ועדשים ודחן וכסמים ונתתה אותם בכלי אחד ועשית אותם לך ללחט…)
> (ואתה קח־לך חטין ושערים ופול).
> —EZEKIEL 4:9, AMP

In the text we see an amazing revelation from the Bible cure. Each specific food contained in the bread mentioned in Ezekiel 4:9 has particular benefits for our health and for preventing disease. Of course, God knew this, and He provided us this wonderful bread for our health and healing.

Here are just a few scientific findings about these food items:

- *Wheat and spelt lower risk for heart disease.* Be sure you use whole wheat, including the bran and germ—not refined wheat. Whole wheat is an excellent source of B complex vitamins, phosphorus, iron, and vitamin E. The vitamin E in wheat helps the body reduce the production of free radicals (which cause LDL cholesterol to stick to artery walls), thus reducing the risk of heart disease. The fiber in wheat helps to reduce the risk of colon cancer.

- *Barley also helps to lower your risk of heart disease.* Do your arteries a favor by eating both wheat and barley. Barley can help lower cholesterol, reduce the formation of blood clots, improve digestion, and reduce the risk of certain forms of cancer. It fights heart disease in two ways: The tocopherols in barley help to stop free radical oxidation, a process that makes LDL cholesterol (the dangerous type) stick to artery walls. They also help to prevent tiny blood clots from forming. Because barley is high in selenium and vitamin E, it helps protect and fight against cancer.

- *Beans (pinto, lentils, kidney, great northern, and others) help lower cholesterol and are packed with soluble fiber.* They can also help to stabilize blood sugar levels, reduce the risk of breast and prostate cancers, and lower the risk of heart disease in people with diabetes.

- *Millet and spelt can help to ease premenstrual discomfort and to speed healing in wounds.* Millet contains protein, which helps the body build and repair muscles, connective fibers, and other tissues.

## לֶחֶם — *Bread*

Because the Bible portrays ordinary people in the round of daily life, *bread* is a common word in its pages, from the first mention in Genesis 3:19. Every day was baking day in the homes of Palestine. Barley or wheat flour was mixed with water and salt, then baked in simple ovens. The loaves produced were such a staple of the diet that bread and food are sometimes interchangeable terms. (See Genesis 37:25; Judges 13:16; Proverbs 27:27.) When, in judgment, God threatened to break the people's "staff of bread," the very basis of their lives was imperiled. (See Leviticus 26:26.) Conversely, when God promised them "a land wherein thou shalt eat bread without scarceness," it was the promise of life itself (Deut. 8:9). This virtual identification of bread with existence led biblical authors to speak metaphorically about the bread of anxious toil (Ps. 127:2, AMP), of wickedness (Prov. 4:17), of idleness (Prov. 31:27), and of tears (Ps. 80:5).

Bread also occupied a significant place in the religious lives of biblical people. The sacrificial system included cereal offerings (Lev. 2:4, AMP). Both tabernacle and temple required the permanent display of showbread, or "bread of the Presence" (Exod. 25:30, AMP; 1 Chron. 28:16). The festival of unleavened bread lay at the heart of Israel's remembrance of the Exodus. Equally linked with God's protective and providential activity was the provision of manna, the "bread from heaven" that sustained Israel's life in the wilderness (Exod. 16:4).

In the Gospels, Jesus acknowledged the importance of bread by quoting Deuteronomy 8:3, "Man doth not live by bread only," and then He identified Himself as the true bread from heaven that gives life to the world. (See Matthew 4:4; Luke 4:4; John 6:33.) At the Last Supper, He interpreted the breaking of the unleavened bread of Passover as symbolizing the offering of Himself, and this ceremonial act was commemorated by early Christians in the ceremony of the "breaking of bread" (Acts 2:42).[2]

## EZEKIEL BREAD, A RECIPE FROM THE OLD TESTAMENT*

2½ cups whole wheat
1½ cups whole rye
½ cup barley
¼ cup millet

$^{1}/_{4}$ cup lentils
2 Tbsp. great northern beans (uncooked)
2 Tbsp. red kidney beans (uncooked)
2 Tbsp. pinto beans (uncooked)
2 cups lukewarm water, divided
$^{1}/_{2}$ cup plus 1 tsp. honey, divided
2 Tbsp. yeast
$^{1}/_{4}$ cup extra-virgin olive oil

Measure and combine all the dry ingredients, except the yeast, in a large bowl. Put this mixture into a flour mill and grind. The flour should be the consistency of regular flour. Coarse flour may cause digestion problems. This makes eight cups of flour. Use four cups per batch of bread.

Measure four cups of flour into a large bowl. Store the remaining flour mixture in the freezer for future use.

Measure one cup lukewarm water (110–115 degrees) in a small mixing bowl. Add 1 teaspoon of the honey and the yeast, stir to dissolve the yeast, cover, and set aside, allowing the yeast to rise for five to ten minutes.

In a small mixing bowl, combine the following: olive oil, $^{1}/_{2}$ cup honey, and remaining cup of warm water. Mix well and add this to the flour mixture in the large bowl. Add the yeast to the bowl and stir until well mixed. The mixture should be the consistency of slightly "heavy" cornbread. Spread the mixture evenly in a 11- by 15-inch pan sprayed with no-cholesterol cooking oil. Let the mixture rise for one hour in a warm place.

Bake at 375 degrees for approximately thirty minutes. Check for doneness. Bread should be the consistency of baked cornbread.

If a flour mill is not available for your use, Ezekiel flour can be ordered from a baking catalog or through a health food store. If such flours are used, however, the texture of the bread will be entirely different from the above recipe.

* This recipe has been adapted directly from Ezekiel 4:9.

# 6

# The Bible Cure:
# Practical Steps You Can Take

THE FOODS IN the Bible cure's Mediterranean Diet abound
with natural substances created by God to aid in protecting us from the ravages of disease. In a spiritual sense, the
Bible frequently speaks of God's placing a hedge of protection around His people. מסביב מעשׂה ידיו ברכת ומקנהו פרץ בארץ
הלא־את שׂכת בעדו ובעד־ביתו ובעד כל־אשר־לו: Translated, we read:
"Hast not thou made an hedge about him, and about his
house, and about all that he hath on every side? Thou hast
blessed the work of his hands, and his substance is increased
in the land" (Job 1:10). Notice that the hedge is placed about
him as well as about his household and possessions. In other
words, his physical body is protected as well as his material
goods. How does the Bible cure provide for protection of our
bodies through the natural part of our pathway of healing?

## BALANCING THE IMMUNE SYSTEM

THE BIBLE CURE'S "natural" hedge of protection inside the

human body protects us from a vast onslaught of diseases and illnesses. This natural hedge is known as the *immune system.* This incredible system protects us from anything from the "sniffles" of a cold to the destruction of cancer. An over-reactive immune system can attack our own body cells, resulting in diseases such as lupus and rheumatoid arthritis (auto-immune diseases). A failure of the immune system can result in cancer, and an overly sensitive immune system can result in allergies. A weakened immune system accelerates the aging process.

Science has begun to discover a fascinating array of natural substances that actually strengthen the immune system. It turns out that God has already provided substances in the plant kingdom to enhance our immune function. We have now been able to concentrate these substances, and we can use them to build up our "hedge of protection" to fight off many diseases and illnesses.

The following twelve natural substances help us to balance and protect our immune systems:

1. *Vitamin E*—helps to preserve and strengthen the immune system function. A weakened immune system can be helped by taking vitamin E in natural form, using a dosage of 800 IU daily.

2. *Multiple vitamins*—a simple multiple-vitamin capsule (such as Theragran-M) is essential to maintain a complete balance in a normal immune system. Take one daily.

3. *B Complex*—$B_{100}$ Complex contains all the various B vitamins. $B_6$ has demonstrated a particularly strong positive effect on the immune system and is found in $B_{100}$ Complex.

4. *Vitamin C*—this vitamin has an important role in increasing the number of white blood cells that form the backbone of our immune response. Take

1,000 milligrams of vitamin C twice daily. Do not use a timed-release capsule.

5. *Zinc*—has long been known as an important substance in protecting the immune system. Too much, however, can cause harmful effects; 15 to 30 milligrams daily is sufficient (the amount found in most multiple vitamin pills).

6. *Chromium*—has an indirect effect on the immune system by stimulating T-lymphocytes and interferon. Take 200 micrograms daily.

7. *Yogurt*—the live cultures in yogurt stimulate the immune system by causing the body to increase production of gamma interferon, which can fight off infections; one to two cups daily is recommended.

8. *Coenzyme Q-10 (Co Q-10)*—studies show that this enzyme can increase an important component of the immune system (gamma globulin). A dosage of 30 milligrams daily is recommended as maintenance therapy; 90 milligrams are recommended if a disease is present.

9. *Garlic*—can stimulate and enhance the response of the immune system. Take the capsule form, equivalent to one clove of fresh garlic daily.

10. *Selenium*—can enhance the immune system function, especially in fighting cancer. It can, however, be toxic in high dosages, so limit the dosage to 100 micrograms daily.

11. *Echinacea*—this plant substance can also stimulate immune system function. It should not be taken daily as a tolerance can develop, making it less effective. Take two to three teaspoons of tincture daily (or

you can take the capsules) for four to eight weeks; then stop taking it for two weeks.

12. *Glutathione*—a potent antioxidant and immune-system stimulant; a standard dosage is 100 milligrams daily.

## OTHER VITAMINS AND ANTIOXIDANTS

IN MATTHEW 24, Jesus describes several events that will occur in the last days. In Matthew 24:7, He specifically notes pestilences or diseases: "there shall be…pestilences.…" Many of the diseases we will see in the last days (AIDS, for example) attack our immune system. We must, therefore, take measures to be certain we fortify the immune system and strengthen it as much as possible.

Researchers have identified many substances that can strengthen the immune system and decrease the occurrence of many forms of cancer and heart disease. One such group is known as antioxidants. These include vitamin C, vitamin E, beta carotene, and selenium.

There are many different food sources for the antioxidants we need. The following list names some of these sources:

- *Vitamin C*—citrus fruits, strawberries, cantaloupe, broccoli, potatoes, tomatoes, and other fruits

- *Vitamin E*—vegetable oils (olive, canola), wheat germ, whole-grain bread, and pasta

- *Beta carotene*—broccoli, cantaloupe, carrots, spinach, squash, pumpkin, sweet potatoes, apricots, and other dark green, orange, and yellow vegetables

- *Selenium*—fish, meat, breads, and cereals

Another substance that seems to have a strong protective effect on numerous body functions is the trace mineral *chromium.* Found in brewers yeast, whole-wheat products, wheat bran, apple peel, and other substances, chromium plays a role in diabetes, cholesterol levels, heart disease, and cataracts; it may be involved in the aging process itself.

## SUPPLEMENT DOSAGES

TO ENSURE AN adequate intake of vitamins and minerals, many people take supplements. Based on current information, you will find listed below the supplements I take and those recommended by many researchers. Take these after a meal.

- Vitamin C, 1,000 milligrams twice daily

- Vitamin E, 800 IU once daily (natural form)

- Beta carotene, 15 milligrams once daily. Beta carotene may come in dosages of 25,000 IU, which equals 15 milligrams. Smokers should not take this supplement.

- Selenium, 100 micrograms once daily

- Chromium picolinate, 200 micrograms once daily

- Coenzyme Q-10 (Co Q-10), 30 milligrams once daily

- $B_{100}$ Complex, one tablet daily

- Garlic, the equivalent of one clove daily

- Multiple vitamins (such as Theragran-M or equivalent), once daily

- Calcium (carbonate), 1,000 milligrams once daily

The above recommendations are for adults and children above the age of sixteen. Children ages sixteen and under should use a multipurpose children's vitamin.

## IMPROVING MEMORY AND MENTAL FUNCTION

SECOND TIMOTHY 1:7 says, "God hath not given us the spirit of fear; but of power, and of love, and of a sound mind." The Word of God renews our mind in a spiritual sense, but the question arises as to whether God can, through physical means (such as food), also cause changes in the mental realm. He said that He would "take sickness away from the midst," but His blessing first had to be on our food (Exod. 23:25). Indeed, we have discovered that foods can have a significant affect on mood, memory, and other mental functions. Some of these foods are listed below:

1. *Fish*—For years fish has been termed a "brain food." In fact, seafood is high in selenium, and studies have determined that people who do not get enough selenium in their bodies tend to suffer more depression, fatigue, and anxiety. When enough selenium is available, mood changes improve significantly. A daily dose of 100 micrograms is often recommended to assure adequate intake (and to provide a cancer protective effect).

2. *Nuts*—Certain nuts (Brazil nuts, walnuts) are high in selenium and can elevate mood. Sunflower seeds and oat bran are also high in selenium.

3. *Folic acid*—A deficiency of folic acid can lead to depression, dementia, and even psychiatric problems. Folate (folic acid) deficiency is common in the United States, and studies show that correcting folic-acid deficiency with as little as 400 micrograms daily can increase brain chemical transmitters (serotonin) and can correct forgetfulness, depression, and irritability. Good sources are spinach (one cup cooked), lima beans, and green leafy vegetables

(or a supplement of 400 micrograms daily).

4. *Garlic*—Studies indicate that garlic tends to be a mood elevator. People who take it regularly report less irritability, fatigue, and anxiety. We recommend that you consider a daily concentrated capsule equivalent to one clove. (Garlic has heart-protective and cancer-preventive effects as well.)

5. *Peppers*—Capsaicin, a primary chemical in chili peppers, can cause the release of brain chemicals (endorphins) that produce increases in mood and feelings.

6. *Caffeine*—Caffeine is a widely used mood elevator taken by literally millions of people. Studies show it can indeed function as a mild antidepressant through a complex effect on certain brain chemicals. Additional studies indicate that caffeine can actually increase concentration as well as reaction times and thought processes. Don't exceed two cups of regular coffee daily. It should be avoided by individuals with a history of irregular heartbeats, fibrocystic breast changes, and other medical problems.

A major concern to many of our patients as they get older is their memory. Though forgetting names and such things is not unusual, we need to identify the natural ways God gave us to keep our minds strong. Six different substances have emerged in recent research that are important to proper memory function.

1. *Zinc*—Slight deficiencies in zinc can lead to poor memory function and mental activity in general. Regular intake of cereals, turkey, and legumes (all high in zinc) can prevent deficiencies. The amount of zinc in most multiple vitamins (15 milligrams) is generally sufficient to supply our needs.

2. *Beta Carotene*—Adequate amounts are critical to ensure proper thought processes. Good sources are dark green leafy vegetables, carrots, and sweet potatoes. One 15-milligram capsule daily can supply more than enough (and offer cancer and heart protection).

3. *Iron*—Essential to maintain normal mental functions, iron is found in greens, lean red meat, and in multiple vitamins—although excessive amounts can be harmful.

4. *Riboflavin*—Found in almonds (ten per day), cereals, and fat-free milk, riboflavin is helpful in maintaining memory function.

5. *Thiamine*—Another essential substance for normal memory function, thiamine is found in wheat bran cereal, nuts (e.g. almonds), and wheat germ.

6. *Avoid animal fat*—Animal fat not only increases the risk of heart disease and numerous cancers, but it also alters chemical transmitters in the brain that in turn can cause memory changes and affect thought processes. Eat lean beef no more than once weekly. Remember: Use fat-free milk and fat-free cheeses. Limit butter, margarine, and sweets, and remove the skin from chicken. (See Leviticus 3:17; 7:23.)

## USING HERBAL MEDICINES

THERE IS A rapidly growing interest in what is known as "alternative medicine"—medical practices that vary from the traditional. One such area involves the use of herbs. Are herbs safe? Which ones are being studied and used the most? This section will explore this area of medical practice. Certain insurance companies are now paying for herbal treatments if prescribed by a doctor, and even the FDA is studying and encouraging research into the use of herbal preparations.

Up to 50 percent of our current prescription medicines originated from the plant kingdom. Powerful chemicals exist within plants—many can help us; some can harm us.

There are many herbs that pose definite dangers. But the problem is that many herbal ingredients simply have not been studied very much. We do know, for example, that comfrey, coltsfoot, and borage contain toxins (pyrrolizidine alkaloids) that taken over time can cause liver damage. Chaparral can also cause liver failure. Pennyroyal, yohimbe, kola nut, and mahuang can also lead to medical problems.

Let's look at the thirteen best-selling herbs to see what has been learned about them.

1. *Chamomile*—used as a tea, ointment, and lotion, and even as a mild sedative. It also seems to be effective in treating inflammation and spasms in the digestive track.

2. *Echinacea*—has been shown to stimulate the immune system and is used for colds and flu-like infections. Only use intermittently (eight weeks maximum); the tincture preparation is strongest. Two to three teaspoons are recommended as a daily dosage.

3. *Feverfew*—the most promising use for feverfew has been in the treatment of headaches, particularly migraines. It is also used for arthritis and stomach pain. Use the dry leaves (25 milligrams twice daily), or the fluid extract (one-fourth to one-half teaspoon three times daily).

4. *Garlic*—has demonstrated multiple benefits. It fights bacteria, strengthens the immune system, raises the good (HDL) cholesterol, and has potent cancer-fighting effects. Dried capsules equivalent to one clove of fresh garlic daily is suggested.

5. *Ginger*—used to prevent nausea and motion sickness and for digestion. It may help to fight colds. One gram of powdered root is typically used two to three times daily.

6. *Ginkgo (biloba)*—has been shown in many studies to improve circulation, especially to the brain, and therefore may improve short term memory loss and headaches; it also may be beneficial in depression. Ginkgo functions as an antioxidant also. A typical dose is 40 milligrams three times daily.

7. *Ginseng*—has been recommended for increasing physical and mental capacities and for times of stress to build up the body's resistance. The data on ginseng is not as convincing as many other herbs, and there is much abuse in marketing this herb. More involved studies are currently in progress.

8. *Goldenseal*—a tea used for respiratory problems and sinusitis. It may fight certain bacterial and parasitic infections, but should not be taken for long periods of time (two weeks at a time maximum). Dosage would be a cup of tea (2 to 4 grams) three times daily, or use the tincture, taking one and one-half to three teaspoons three times daily.

9. *Milk thistle*—has been used in Europe to treat cirrhosis of the liver; it helps liver cells rejuvenate in conditions such as jaundice or inflammation of the liver cells due to the effects of the chemical silymarin. A standardized extract (70 to 210 milligrams) three times daily has been used.

10. *Peppermint*—has been used for improving digestion, especially excessive gas. It is usually used as a tea, but exact beneficial dosage is not known.

11. *Saw palmetto*—this plant (*seronoa repens*) has been extensively used in Europe to treat enlarged prostate glands in men. Men experiencing difficulty in urination, slowness, or increased frequency should, of course, consult their doctor, but they might want to try 160 milligrams twice daily.

12. *Valerian*—may be useful as a minor tranquilizer and for sleep disorders. It can be taken as a tea (1 to 2 grams) thirty minutes before retiring, or use the fluid extract (one-half to one teaspoon) or solid extract (250 to 500 milligrams).

13. *Willowbark*—widely used as a tea for headaches, fever, muscular pains, and arthritis. Contains salicylates, the active ingredient in aspirin. Probably too weak an herb to be useful; coated aspirin would be more effective.

These natural substances are all part of the Bible cure's pathway of health. In this chapter so far we have discussed their use as part of a daily nutritional diet to help the body build up a resistance to diseases of many kinds. In the remainder of the chapter we are going to look more closely at some of the characteristics of these natural substances that actually help our bodies to effect healing from a number of diseases.

## HEALING ARTHRITIS

ONE OF THE most common, painful, and debilitating diseases facing men and women is arthritis, specifically osteoarthritis. There are many forms of arthritis (such as rheumatoid arthritis, gouty arthritis, and others). In osteoarthritis, the most common form, the cartilage between joints softens and becomes thinner, and the cartilage breaks down and becomes less elastic. This process can be detected on x-rays in nearly everyone over the age of forty, but one may not have pain from it (although fifteen to twenty million Americans do). Symptoms include pain in the knuckles, big toes, thumbs, hips, knees, upper and lower spine, and stiffness, especially in the morning.

What can you do to slow down this process and keep bone from rubbing against bone as the cartilage becomes thinner? There are several techniques we can follow; some are well-known and well-tested, while others are much newer with fewer formal studies but with strong suggestive evidence of effectiveness.

The following treatments represent the latest methods that seem to be working to relieve the pain and swelling of osteoarthritis and to keep the disease from worsening.

1. *Glucosamine*—This substance (an amino sugar) is produced naturally in the body, but it can be purchased without a prescription. It stimulates cartilage repair and is anti-inflammatory. A typical dosage would be 500 milligrams three times daily. It is available in health food stores and is very safe to take.

2. *Chondroitin sulfate*—This chemical, which is produced in the body (also an amino sugar), helps increase water retention in the cartilage, making it more elastic. It also blocks enzymes that destroy cartilage. A typical dosage is 1,000 to 2,000 milligrams daily; this may also be obtained at a health food store and is also very safe to take.

3. *Vitamin D*—A study from Boston University Medical Center showed that vitamin D can keep osteoarthritis from advancing, especially in the knees. This vitamin helps keep the cartilage intact and helps prevent deterioration of the bones. The dosage recommended is 400 units daily (too high a dosage can cause liver problems).

4. *Exercise*—Exercise actually nourishes joints. Bearing down or exercising a joint "stirs up" nutrients in the cartilage; movements cause the fluid to flow back

into cartilage. This process can both nourish and lubricate the joints. Brisk walking, water aerobics, and stationary cycling are all good anti-arthritis exercises.

5. *Body weight*—This is one of the most important areas to address; too much weight on your frame will literally wear out the cartilage. If you are ready to reduce, get our *Techniques for Weight Loss* study guide (#215-S) and *The Mediterranean Diet* (God's ideal diet for today) study guide (#222-S.). Some of our patients have lost as much as sixty pounds by following these study guides.

6. *Manage pain*—Hot showers, baths, and hot packs stimulate circulation and relieve pain. The occasional use of Tylenol can be helpful, but do not take it daily—it can affect the kidneys in some people. Also be careful with ibuprofen, aspirin, and naproxen as they can affect the stomach and kidneys.

7. *Other treatments*—Certain herbs can help with arthritis, but studies are sparse. Capsaicin (an ointment from cayenne peppers) can block pain. Ginger (powdered ginger root) has been reported to help many individuals at doses of 1,000 to 3,000 milligrams per day. Both of these are available from pharmacies or health food stores. One final word of caution: Consult with a physician to be sure what kind of arthritis you have. The above recommendations are for the "wear-and-tear" type of osteoarthritis. Rheumatoid arthritis (a less common form of arthritis) is an overreaction of the immune system (order our *Balancing the Immune System* study guide, #87-S). Other forms of arthritis, such as gout, require entirely different treatments (you should see your doctor).

Remember: In order to pray the "effectual and fervent prayer of a righteous man" (James 5:16), you need to know specifically the kind of arthritis you are fighting in order to take authority over it. Always combine the spiritual power of prayer with the natural methods described above to obtain your pathway to healing.

## HEALING DIABETES

DIABETES IS A major health problem affecting as many as fifteen million Americans with five hundred thousand new cases each year. Diabetes can affect the heart, eyes, kidneys, and nerves. The exciting news is that there are newly discovered techniques that can lower blood sugar and may even reverse diabetes. Fiber is turning out to be a major factor used to lower blood sugar. Fiber has decreased insulin requirements 30 to 40 percent in Type I diabetics. In Type II diabetes, most patients were off insulin in ten to twenty days in one study.

What are the keys to lowering diabetic risks and possibly reversing it?

- *Water-soluble fiber*—obtained from oat bran (one-third cup daily); dried beans (one-half cup five times weekly); including kidney, pinto, and great northern beans; psyllium (one to three teaspoons daily).

- *Fish*—in a study carried out over four years, 45 percent of nonfish eaters developed glucose intolerance versus only 25 percent of the fish eaters. Fish eaters were only half as likely to get glucose intolerance as nonfish eaters. Eating as little as one ounce of fish four to five times weekly was sufficient. Try to eat cold-water fish such as cod, salmon, mackerel, and trout.

- *Exercise*—of twenty-two thousand people in one study, those who exercised five or more times weekly had only 42 percent of the incidence of diabetes compared to those who exercised less than once weekly. Those exercising two to four times a week had 38 percent of the incidence of diabetes compared to those who exercised less than once weekly. Even those who exercised only once weekly had only 23 percent as high an incidence of diabetes as those who exercised less than once weekly.

- *Vitamins and minerals*—certain vitamins such as the antioxidants (vitamins C, E, beta carotene, and selenium) may offer some protection to the arteries in persons who have diabetes. Diabetics should take 800 to 1,000 micrograms of chromium picolinate daily. (Order our vitamin study guide (#211-S) if you would like more details.)

## Reversing Heart Disease

Over 53 percent of people in large industrialized countries die of heart disease. It is caused by fat deposits that build up in the arteries, often beginning in the teenage years. Symptoms range from angina (tightness or pressure in the chest) to the severe pain associated with a heart attack to congestive heart failure with fluid accumulation in the body. The following steps can be used to reverse heart disease if you have it and to prevent it if you are currently free of problems.

1. *Reduce fat intake*—Eat beef no more than three to four times per month and no meat at all three days per week. Eat only fruit and vegetables on these days. Eat fish at least two to three times per week, preferably cold-water fish (salmon, cod, herring). Use canola and olive oil.

2. *Exercise*—A minimum of three times per week and a maximum of six times per week is a good schedule. Exercise for thirty to sixty minutes per session. Do the entire time of exercise at one time, and keep your heart rate up, not allowing it to fall. Walking, cycling, stationary cycling, indoor track

machine, and jogging are all good forms of exercise.

3. *Vitamins*—Take your recommended vitamins, especially vitamin E (800 units per day). It may keep LDL (the bad cholesterol) from depositing in your arteries.

4. *Coenzyme Q-10 (Co Q-10)*—A minimum dosage of 30 milligrams per day is appropriate; more (100 mg.) can be taken with certain types of heart problems (congestive heart failure); check with your doctor.

5. *Garlic*—Take one or two concentrated capsules daily. Strengths vary, but the equivalent of one clove daily thins blood and may raise HDL "good" cholesterol.

6. *Bran*—Include water-soluble bran in your daily eating plan. We recommend one-third cup of oat bran daily and an additional form of wheat bran such as All Bran or Fiber One cereal (one-half cup daily).

7. *Psyllium*—Take one to two teaspoons daily if your cholesterol is high.

8. *A low-salt diet*—Find ways to reduce your salt intake—use no added salt when your foods are prepared, and use "lite salt" or salt substitute at the table.

9. *Lose weight*—Begin following the guidelines of *The Bible Cure* to take off the unnecessary and detrimental pounds. Weigh once weekly, and lose two to three pounds per week—no more, no less. If you haven't lost that amount, reduce your calories the following week until you do. Eat breakfast and a "light" evening meal.

10. *Baby aspirin*—Take one daily (81 mg., coated), but check with a doctor; some people should not take aspirin.

11. *Control blood pressure*—It is imperative to control your blood pressure. If your new Bible cure eating plan still does not keep your blood pressure down, ask your doctor if you need a prescription to help. There are new one-pill-per-day drugs that work great. These medicines control blood pressure without side effects (ACE inhibitors, calcium channel blockers).

12. *Control blood sugar*—Get your blood sugar checked. If your blood sugar is high, there are simple ways to lower it. See our study guide (#212-S) on diabetes if this is a problem.

13. *Get regular checkups*—Know what you're battling against; get a regular stress test (walking electrocardiograms), blood work, and a good head-to-toe checkup.

14. *Get cholesterol down*—If the above measures don't work to lower your cholesterol, ask your doctor about the new once-daily medicines derived from plants that can lower blood fats. These drugs cause almost no side effects and can reverse hardening in arteries, but they must be given by a doctor. Get your total cholesterol under two hundred, the cholesterol to HDL ratio under four, and the LDL cholesterol to one hundred.

15. *Treat your symptoms*—If you have angina (chest pain, tightness, pressure), some of the new medications (calcium channel blockers) can actually reverse hardening of the arteries.

16. *Congestive heart failure*—The new ACE inhibitors

are essential for this disease. If you have congestive heart failure, you must restrict your salt intake to three grams per day and restrict your fluid intake as well. Take up to 100 milligrams of Co Q-10. Other medicines such as Lanoxin may also be needed.

## HARDENING OF THE ARTERIES

THERE ARE NINE dietary factors that decrease the risk of hardening of the arteries (a condition that can lead to a stroke or heart attack):

1. *Eat more complex carbohydrates* by increasing your intake of fruit, cereal, and vegetables.

2. *Emphasize polyunsaturated fats in your diet,* including olive oil and canola oil, which lower cholesterol levels.

3. *Increase fiber in your diet* (especially oat bran).

4. *Keep your alcohol intake to a minimum*—high amounts of alcohol will increase your blood pressure and risk of stroke.

5. *Limit your caffeine intake to two cups of regular coffee per day.* Remember that caffeine may increase your cholesterol levels and lead to heart irregularities.

6. *Limit salt in your diet*—it may increase blood pressure.

7. *Reduce your cholesterol levels* by limiting your intake of egg yokes, cheeses, and fatty meats.

8. *Lower the amount of saturated fats that you consume*—limit butter, cream, and whole milk (use

fat-free milk), chocolate, pastries, coconut, and palm oil.

9. *Avoid excess calories in your diet*—match your intake of calories to your exercise levels.

## Fighting Cancer

The National Cancer Institute and numerous other research centers are in the midst of great research projects on chemicals in foods (phytochemicals) that can prevent, and perhaps even counter, the effects of cancer in the body. Interestingly, thirty-five centuries ago God told us about food. He felt the issue of our diet was so important that He created the world, animals, and man in the space of the first twenty-eight verses of Genesis—reserving the last half of chapter one to talk about food. Approximately one person in five will die of cancer (roughly fifteen hundred people per day), but some estimates indicate that up to 50 or 60 percent of all cancer cases could be prevented with better nutrition.

### Ten Foods That Fight Cancer

Researchers are discovering numerous anticancer compounds in foods. Some prevent a cell from developing into malignancy while others tend to block the blood supply to the cancer. There are ten different classes of foods that are showing particular promise. The following list will give you a quick reference to these.

1. *Soybeans*—Soybeans contain genistein, which may cut off the blood supply to cancer cells. It may be especially helpful for breast and ovarian cancer as it can block certain estrogen receptors. Choices of foods include tofu, soy flour, and miso. Peanuts, mung beans, and alfalfa sprouts contain lesser amounts of this chemical. Soybeans also contain other strong anti-cancer compounds (protease inhibitors, saponins)

111

that increase immune-system function.

2. *Chili peppers*—A chemical found in peppers, capsaicin, may neutralize certain cancer-causing substances (nitrosamines) and help to prevent cancers such as stomach cancer.

3. *Garlic and onions*—Both of these contain allium compounds (diallyl sulfides), which increase the activity of immune cells that fight cancer and indirectly help to break down cancer-causing substances. Chives also contain this chemical. Over thirty anticancer compounds are present in these substances. Not only can garlic prevent cancer, but it can directly fight cancer (ajoane chemicals) and can stimulate the body's defense mechanisms. Consider dried garlic extract (capsules), taking the equivalent of one clove daily. Eat onions frequently.

4. *Grapes*—Grapes contain ellagic acid. This compound blocks enzymes that are necessary for cancer cells to grow, thus slowing the growth of tumors. Grapes also contain compounds that can prevent blood clots. Another substance in grape skins (resveratrol) prevents the deposit of cholesterol in arteries.

5. *Citrus fruits*—Citrus contains limonene, which stimulates cancer-killing immune cells (T-lymphocytes and others). They also break down cancer-causing substances. Oranges in particular have shown strong anticancer benefits. Some sixty anticancer chemicals are contained in citrus fruits. Limes and celery also fall into this category, though they are less potent.

6. *Licorice root*—A chemical, glycyrrhizin, blocks a component of testosterone and therefore may help to prevent the growth of prostate cancer. This is

found in the root of licorice (not the candy form). Caution: Excessive amounts can lead to elevated blood pressure.

7. *Tomatoes*—Tomatoes contain lycopene, an anti-cancer substance that some researchers suggest may be stronger than beta carotene. Watermelons, carrots, and red peppers also contain this powerful substance. Vitamin C, an antioxidant that can prevent cellular damage leading to cancer, is also found in tomatoes.

8. *Tea (not herbal teas)*—Tea contains certain antioxidants known as polyphenois (catechins), which prevent cancer cells from dividing. Green tea is best, followed by our more common black tea (herbal teas do not show this benefit). Drink two to three glasses daily.

9. *Broccoli and cabbage*—These cruciferous vegetables contain multiple cancer-fighting chemicals (indoles for example). Indoles can affect estrogen, converting it to a benign form that will not stimulate abnormal breast-cancer cells. Brussels sprouts and cauliflower also fall in this category.

10. *Greens*—The darker they are, the more the cancer-fighting chemicals such as lutein, beta carotene, and carotenoids. Spinach and lettuce (dark romaine) are all good sources.

## Decreasing the Risk of Cancer

There are thirteen major dietary factors that affect the risk of cancer. Read these factors carefully, and then determine that you will follow these guidelines to decrease your own risk of developing cancer in your body.

- Increase foods rich in vitamin A in your diet (apricots, cantaloupe, peaches, carrots, pumpkin, sweet potatoes).

- Eat cruciferous vegetables daily (broccoli, Brussels sprouts, cabbage, cauliflower).

- Include foods rich in vitamin C in your diet (cantaloupe, collard greens, cabbage, strawberries, spinach, broccoli, oranges, tomatoes, cauliflower).

- Eat some fiber daily (wheat fiber such as Fiber One and other bran type cereals; oat fiber such as Quaker Oat Bran Cereal).

- Include foods that are rich in selenium (chicken, seafoods, and grains).

- Include foods rich in vitamin E (olive and canola oils, cereals, green leafy vegetables).

- Limit caffeine in your diet. It may increase the incidence of certain cancers (bladder, pancreas).

- Limit your use of artificial sweeteners; limit especially saccharin because we are uncertain of possible cancer effects.

- Avoid heat-charred foods. Be careful with grilled and charcoaled foods—they may increase the risk of cancer.

- Avoid foods containing nitrites such as smoked foods; they may increase the risk of cancer. Limit bacon, hot dogs, sausage, bologna, salami, smoked fish, and smoked lunch meats.

- Avoid excess calories. Too many calories may increase the risk of colon, uterine, and breast cancer.

- Avoid excessive use of alcohol, which may lead to liver,

mouth, throat, and esophageal cancer.

- Decrease the amount of fat in your diet. Fat increases the risk of colon, breast, and prostate cancer—consume very little fat and avoid butter, limit egg yolks, cheese, pastries, and fatty meats.

## If You Have Cancer

If you have cancer, consider the following foods and nutrition guidelines:

1. *Fats*—Decrease, if not eliminate, animal fats. Avoid safflower, corn, and peanut oil. Use more monosaturated fats such as olive oil and canola oil.

2. *Fish oil*—Omega-3 fatty acids in cold-water fish (cod, mackerel, herring) may decrease the size of cancerous tumors. Fish-oil capsules may also be taken.

3. *Beta carotene*—It can not only help to prevent cancer, but it shows promise fighting cancer. Orange and yellow vegetables and fruits are good (sweet potatoes and cantaloupe, for example). Capsules (30 milligrams per day) as a supplement are suggested.

4. *Cabbage, broccoli*—These vegetables are potent cancer fighters, especially breast cancer; eat several portions daily.

5. *Yogurt*—Nonfat yogurt can help the body increase levels of cancer-fighting chemicals; eat six to eight ounces daily.

6. *Licorice*—As we saw earlier, the roots are being studied for cancer-fighting properties. A proper dose is not currently known. The ground root may be made into a tea.

There are other supplements besides the above foods that we recommend for their cancer-fighting properties. To find out about some of these, get our *Vitamins* study guide (#211-S).

## PREVENTING PROSTATE CANCER

PROSTATE CANCER IS now the most common tumor in men. It will strike a quarter million men yearly and kill almost forty thousand men per year. The new blood test (PSA) should be done on all men over age fifty and on men under age fifty who have a family history of prostate cancer. All men should follow the eight steps listed below to help prevent the cancer from forming and to help cure it if you have it.

1. *Decrease saturated fat*—Eat beef no more than three times per month. Avoid cheese and switch to fat-free milk. Red meat is especially linked to increased risk, and butter is also. Avoid mayonnaise, creamy salad dressings, and butter because of a fatty acid (alpha linoleic acid); do use olive oil and canola oil as your main sources of fat.

2. *Antioxidants*—Get plenty of vitamins C, E, and beta carotene from yellow, orange and dark green fruits and vegetables. Almonds (ten per day) can supply vitamin E. Add the following supplements to your daily diet: vitamin C (1,000 milligrams twice daily), vitamin E (800 units daily), beta carotene (30 milligrams or 50,000 units daily).

3. *Calcium*—This can help decrease tumor formation and may decrease uptake of a fatty acid that causes tumor formation (alpha linoleic acid). Get calcium from nonfat yogurt, nonfat cottage cheese, and fat-free milk. Add 1,000 milligrams of calcium (calcium carbonate) daily to your diet.

4. *Garlic*—As we illustrated earlier, the more garlic

people have in their diet, the less their cancer incidence. Garlic can limit tumor growth markedly, kill cancer cells, and shrink tumors. Use a garlic press or take capsules daily that are equivalent to one clove of garlic. It must be taken consistently.

5. *Vitamin D*—High levels of vitamin D can protect from prostate cancer. Men in sunny climates have a lower incidence of prostate cancer (sun causes the skin to make vitamin D, but don't overdo sun exposure). Good sources are fortified fat-free milk and fish. Be careful with supplements—200 units per day can be toxic. Get vitamin D from foods.

6. *Tea*—Compounds in green tea can inhibit tumor growth. Drink two cups per day. Lipton and other companies make green tea.

7. *Soy*—Soy products can limit the spread of cancer and can stop its early growth. Tofu and soy burgers are among the sources of this protective food.

8. *Cumin*—This spice may prevent the development of prostate cancer. It can be used on vegetables and in various dishes.

## PROTECTIVE FOOD SHEET

| | Frequency | Fiber | Cruciferous | Vitamin C | Beta Carotene | Calcium | Omega-3 | Selenium |
|---|---|---|---|---|---|---|---|---|
| Fat-free milk | daily | | | | | H | | |
| Nonfat yogurt | daily | | | | | H | | |
| Whole-wheat bread | daily | H | | | | | | H |
| Oat or wheat bran | daily | H | | | | | | |
| Broccoli | 1 weekly | M | H | H | H | H | | |
| Brussels sprouts | 1 weekly | M | H | H | | | | |
| Cabbage | 1 weekly | M | H | H | | M | | M |
| Cantaloupe | 1 weekly | | | M | M | | | |
| Carrots | 1 weekly | H | | | H | | | M |
| Tomato | 1 weekly | | | M | M | | | |
| Greens (mustard, turnip) | 1 weekly | H | | H | H | M | | |
| Legumes (beans, peas) | 1 weekly | H | | | | M | | |
| Sweet potato | 7–10 days | M | | M | | | | |
| Spinach | 1 weekly | | | M | | | | |
| Strawberries | 1 weekly | M | | H | | | | |
| Lean beef | 1–2 weekly | | | | | | | H |
| Salmon, cod (fresh) | 1 weekly | | | | | | M | M |
| Salmon (canned) | 1 weekly | | | | | M | M | M |
| Tuna (canned) | 1 weekly | | | | | | M | M |

H = High    M=Medium

## BENEFITS OF PHYTOCHEMICALS

| PLANTS | EXTRACTS | HEALTH BENEFITS |
| --- | --- | --- |
| Broccoli, kale, radish | Sulforaphane | Growth deterrent. |
| Cabbage | Isothlocyanate | Lung and other growth deterrent. |
| Cauliflower | Several | Breast growth deterrent. |
| Citrus plants | Quercetin | Allergies and heart problems. |
| Garlic and onion | Allicin | Breaks blood clots, reduces blood pressure, helps normalize high cholesterol levels and irregular heartbeats, deters lung and other growths. |
| Ginger | Gingerol | Arthritis relief, ulcer deterrent, helps heal skin sores and is an antioxidant. |
| Green tea leaves | EGCG | Antioxidant and growth deterrent, reduces cholesterol, helps deter heart problems, strokes, and infections. |
| Ginkgo biloba leaves | Flavones | Improves circulation, reduces blood clots; ameliorates headaches, ringing in the ears, depression, and impotence. |
| Hawthorn plant | Flavonoids | Lowers cholesterol and deters allergies. |
| Paprika | Canthaxanthin | Antioxidant. |
| Rosemary plant | Rosmarinic acid | Deters growths and helps ameliorate heart problems. |
| Spirulina | Several | Detoxifies blood and stimulates production of the body's most powerful antioxidant, superoxide dismutase. |
| Tomato | Lycopenes | Growth and prostate disease deterrent. |
| Turmeric spice plant | Curcumin | Arthritis relief. |
| Various plants | Coumaric acid | Growth deterrent. |
| Most plants | Chlorophyll | Detoxifies blood, helps heal bedsores, and is a growth deterrent. |

# 7

# Facing the Ultimate Cure—
# Death and Beyond

## by Linda Cherry

A N EIGHTY-FOUR-YEAR-OLD woman with many, many complications in her body recently wrote to me, telling me
about the heartache of losing her husband, the grief she faces
daily, and the illnesses her worn-out body is enduring. Near
the end of her letter, she says, "I am not able to go out. I am
in a wheelchair constantly. I am five feet, eight inches tall, and
weigh only one hundred pounds. I cling to the Lord. I am
waiting for Him to take me home. I am preparing myself,
because I want to see Him face to face."

The emphasis of this book is on teaching you the way to
stay healthy. It is to keep you strong in your body so that you
can go fulfill the Great Commission: "Go ye into all the world,
and preach the gospel to every creature" (Mark 16:15). We
teach people that Jesus is the Healer; Jesus is the Deliverer;
Jesus will meet your needs. You are His own. But we must all
prepare to face the moment when God's ultimate cure becomes
ours—when our physical bodies are no longer useful to us
and they die—freeing our spirits to receive our eternal healing

and to see our Great Physician face to face in heaven where we will live eternally.

We all want to hold back the moment of death as long as possible. We want to stay healthy as long as we can, following God's pathway of healing so that He can do in the supernatural what we cannot do in the natural. But the ultimate purpose of our lives—the reason Jesus wants us to give our hearts to Him and become His children—is to prepare for our eternal home.

This is not our home; we are just passing through. The eleventh chapter of Hebrews tells of the "heroes of the faith" who went on to their eternal home:

> These all died in faith, not having received the promises, but having seen them afar off, and were persuaded of them, and embraced them, and confessed that they were strangers and pilgrims on the earth. For they that say such things declare plainly that they seek a country. And truly, if they had been mindful of that country from whence they came out, they might have had opportunity to have returned. But now they desire a better country, that is, an heavenly: wherefore God is not ashamed to be called their God: for he hath prepared for them a city.
>
> —HEBREWS 11:13–16

We, like these early Bible heroes, have been given jobs to do for God on earth. We have been given the great opportunity of having a personal relationship with God, communing with Him, and praising Him daily. We can walk with Him and feel His presence around us. But in the end we all will meet Him face to face. We die a physical death, but we will not die a spiritual death—we will go on and live with Him forever.

When I read letters such as the one above from the eighty-four year old widow, my heart is broken because I feel the pain felt by people who just cannot let go of loved ones that have gone on to be with the Lord. Although they know that their loved one is with the Lord, they struggle for years with letting go.

I recently faced the same struggle. Through the experience

of losing my dad the Lord taught me many things that I believe can be used to help others face such a loss God's way—recognizing death as the ultimate cure for an individual and rejoicing in the release of that loved one from the bondage of a physical body that can no longer support an "abundant life." The Lord was gracious with me, giving me a personal experience with death that can help you to get healing in the areas of your loss.

I have never lost anyone so dear to me as my dad. Dad was diagnosed with brain cancer, and a short five months later he went home to be with the Lord. Those five months were incredible months. Dad and I had many "God talks," as I called them. We shared about the Lord. We reassured each other that Jesus is our Lord and Savior and that we know we will be together in heaven.

It was not the leaving that was the hard part of losing Dad— it was the suffering he endured just before his ultimate cure. I do not know why he had to suffer so long. Perhaps God was allowing all my family members to come to grips with the reality of my dad's imminent departure from this life. Maybe there were some who needed to deal with the question: "What is going to happen to me when I die?" We will never know on this side of eternity why he suffered during those remaining months on earth. That is one of the questions for which I will have no answer until I reach heaven and can talk to God face to face. I have learned to accept the truth in Deuteronomy 29:29 about such questions:

> The secret things belong unto the LORD our God: but those things which are revealed belong unto us and to our children for ever.

One of the "things which are revealed" to me is this: I have treasure in heaven now. Now my dad is in heaven. I have had friends go on to be with the Lord, and I can't wait to see them someday. But heaven has become more real to me; it is a place where I have something so precious—and that knowledge has given me a whole new revelation of heaven.

In 1 Thessalonians 4:13–18 we read:

> And now, brothers and sisters, I want you to know what
> will happen to the Christians who have died so you will
> not be full of sorrow like people who have no hope. For
> since we believe that Jesus died and was raised to life
> again, we also believe that when Jesus comes, God will
> bring back with Jesus all the Christians who have died. I
> can tell you this directly from the Lord: We who are still
> living when the Lord returns will not rise to meet him
> ahead of those who are in their graves. For the Lord him-
> self will come down from heaven with a commanding
> shout, with the call of the archangel, and with the
> trumpet call of God. First, all the Christians who have
> died will rise from their graves. Then, together with them,
> we who are still alive and remain on the earth will be
> caught up in the clouds to meet the Lord in the air and
> remain with him forever. So comfort and encourage each
> other with these words.
>
> —NLT

The Christians who have died are so precious to God that
when Jesus comes again they get to go up first. What a comforting thought for those of us who are grieving over the loss
of a loved one. As we were going through the preparations
for my dad's funeral, I thought of how grief can take a grip on
you unless you take a grip on grief. We are to comfort one
another with these words from 1 Thessalonians 4. We do not
need to mourn and wail as the world mourns and wails. We
have a hope and an assurance in God's love that makes us
strong.

Dad and I talked about many things in the days before his
death. Many times as I sat down beside him he would whisper
quietly, "I want to go home." We talked about heaven, our
eternal home, and what it would be like. Dad had a baby
brother in heaven already who had died very young in his
life, and Dad wanted to see him again. That baby brother had
brought such joy and love into his home. "I want to see him,"

he would tell me. "I want to see Teddy Dale" (that was his name).

"Daddy, you are going to see him," I would reply, and he would get a smile on his face.

It was tragic to see what the brain cancer did to Dad's mind. He always had a brilliant mind; he had a master's degree, was a CPA, and had a very logical, reasoning mind. But he gradually lost the ability to concentrate or to form his thoughts clearly. One of the last rational things he said to me one day as I knelt by his bed was, "Linda, I am tired, and I want to go home, but I don't know how to get there."

"Well, Daddy," I gently responded, "how do we get anything that we want?"

His spirit man knew the answer, but he could not get the right words out. He looked at me and said, "I don't know."

He did know, but he just couldn't think, so I said, "Well, Daddy, we pray. Let's pray about it." So we prayed. When a Christian who is suffering with a devastating illness doesn't want to stay around and suffer any more, they will often express a desire to go home. Their Father is calling them to the place where there is no pain, no sorrow, and no tears.

So I knelt beside my daddy's bed and I prayed, "Father, in the name of Jesus, I ask You to take my daddy home. It is the desire of his heart. He wants to see You, Father. You said You would give us the desires of our hearts, so I am asking You to take him and to grant this desire. We thank You for it, in Jesus' name." Then I said, "Daddy, is that what you wanted?" He shook his head yes, he smiled, and he went to sleep.

Daddy fell into a semicoma and then into a coma. I want to tell you something about people who are in a coma as they get ready to pass into eternity. There have been books written about the testimonies of people who were in comas, and had been given up to die, who came out of the comas. Many have related the fact that they heard the conversations that were taking place in the room as they lay in the coma. Often they will repeat the things that they heard. Some people have said, "I heard you planning my funeral." I know that any of us would feel great despair knowing that a loved one who was lying before us in a coma could hear us discussing the details of his or her funeral!

It is important to remember that even though a person may be in a coma, unable to speak, with the mind not functioning as it should, his spirit man is still alive. As a believer, you can speak to that person's spirit man. At that point you have a great advantage. When I visited my father as he lay in a coma, the Lord quickened that opportunity to me. I had the privilege of speaking to his spirit man even though he could not speak to me.

Every day that I could, I made it a point to go to my dad, kneel down beside his bed so that I could speak right into his ear, and tell him how precious he was to Jesus. "Daddy, you're going home soon," I would say. "Jesus is ready to meet you... He has His arms outstretched to greet you. Daddy, Jesus is going to hold you and hug you and tell you how much He loves you. You are not going to hurt any more."

Sometimes I would say, "Daddy, Jesus loves Jack" (Jack was Daddy's name). "He is waiting for you. You are almost home, Daddy. You are almost home. Angels are coming soon. They are preparing the way. They are going to come and show you how to get there." I took advantage of that opportunity because I knew he could hear me.

Daddy had already made peace with all the people in his life—his brothers and sisters, my brother and sister, and me. He had said things to each one of us that he wanted us to know. He told us how special we were to him... how proud he was of us... how much he loved us. God was so gracious to allow us to hear those words from the man we loved so much, to experience those feelings, and to exchange our love. That love is solid forever until we see Daddy again in heaven.

God is the orchestrator of all events—and this was so evident during these last days with my dad. Above all else, I wanted to be with my dad as he passed from this earth to his eternal home. I had asked the Lord to show me when it would be time for Daddy to go home. I knew that was a bold move, but I prayed: "Father, Jesus doesn't even know when He is coming back to earth to get us, but You know. I know that You and Jesus both know when my daddy is coming to see You. So I am asking You to reveal the time to me. I know it's the season of his passing now, but please reveal to me the time. I am asking in faith, in Jesus' name."

I had not gone to the office or worked as a nurse for several weeks before Dad's death. But on the Monday that Dad died I had to go to work. I had seen some patients, but all of a sudden I looked at my husband and our head nurse, and I said, "I have to go. I have to go right now."

I had an urgency that I should drop everything and get to Mom and Dad's house. (Daddy wanted to die at home, and with the help of wonderful hospice care and lots of Christian visiting nurses that had been possible.) When I reached his bedside, I noticed that his breathing had changed drastically. Immediately, I called my sister. While I was on the phone, I heard his breathing change, so I hung the phone up quickly and went to the side of the bed. Mother was sitting in a chair talking to the nurse. I said, "Mother, you had better come quickly." She came to his left side, and I stood to his right. "Mother, hold his hand," I suggested, and I held his other hand. In another moment his breathing stopped, and Daddy left this world.

I just sat there holding Daddy's hand. As I had tried to prepare myself for this moment, I had thought in the natural that when it came to this point I would just fall apart—just wail and weep and go to pieces. But it was so different. I just sat there thinking, *Here I am holding Daddy's hand. But this body is but a vessel of clay that housed his spirit while he was on earth. He is already in glory.* I had to resist smiling and laughing aloud as my spirit rejoiced, knowing that his pain was gone. The suffering was gone. I knew that Daddy was in glory land, standing before Jesus face to face. It was an awesome moment!

As the family came, and we made all the arrangements for the funeral, I kept remembering the thing that I said to Daddy right before he left...before his breathing changed. I could tell that it was close, and I bent down to his ear like I had for days and said, "Daddy, you are almost home...you are almost home! The angels are coming; you are going to be safe."

Daddy had not responded to anything I said to him in a long time, but all of a sudden his right hand reached up. I just knew that he was reaching up for God to pull him on into heaven, because shortly after that he went on to be with the Lord. It was just such a beautiful moment.

God also had some special revelations that helped me get through the funeral. In the time before the funeral, for some reason I picked up the dictionary and looked up the word *cemetery*. Cemeteries have always been something that I didn't like because, frankly, dead people are there. But when I looked up the word cemetery in the Greek, I discovered that it means "a sleeping chamber...a burial place...to sleep." For those of you who are familiar with cemeteries...people are buried facing east—believers and unbelievers alike. I was reminded of the fact that when Jesus splits the eastern sky, the dead in Christ will rise first...out of their sleeping chamber where they are asleep, awaiting that day.

Another word that always bothered me was the word *casket*. I hate that word. I have always hated that word. So I looked it up, too; it means, "a small chest or box...usually ornamental and lined...a rectangular box or chest for a corpse to be buried in."

I started thinking about that definition—and I still did not like the word very well. But suddenly the Lord put in my spirit the revelation that the chest is a treasure chest holding a precious treasure, asleep until the day of the Rapture. In His Word, God reveals this treasure is so special that the dead will rise first from their treasure chest to meet Him in the air. Only then will we be caught up with them in the air.

These intimate revelations enabled me to face my dad's funeral with joy and hope. The Lord has given me such joy in knowing that he is in the glory and presence of the Lord. I am praying for those of you who are holding on to grief that has bound you in a type of bondage. You may feel the pain of your loss day in and day out. I hope that the example of how God ministered to me through the events of the death of my father will be comforting to you.

I want you to realize for yourself that this earth is not your home. We are just passing through. Pray that when you finish your race, the Lord Jesus will say, "Well done, thou good and faithful servant." Live in the hope of spending eternity with the precious treasures—the loved ones—who have gone on before. Oh, what a day that will be!

# Conclusion

# Finish the Course
# With Joy

I OFTEN ASK PATIENTS, "If God heals you, what are you going to do for God? What is your remaining course if you receive your Bible cure?" Paul talked about finishing the course with joy. He also indicated that his greatest joy would be to be with Jesus for eternity. We all look toward that blessed hope of entering eternity with our Lord and Savior, Jesus Christ. But, we are not ready to enter eternity until the Lord has spoken the final word into our lives, "Well done, good and faithful servant."

As you seek your Bible cure, ask yourself, "What does God have left for me to do in loving and serving Him and others?" Each Christian has a ministry, a special and unique way in which he or she is gifted to serve the Lord.

Are you willing to ask the final question: "When my course is finished with joy, am I ready to pass through the sleep of death and enter into eternal life with God?" Jesus reveals that death is not the end but simply sleeping. (See Mark 5:39; 1 Thessalonians 4:13.) It is simply the way we pass from this life

131

into eternal life (John 3:16; 1 John 5:20).

If you do not know Jesus as your personal Lord and Savior, I invite you right now to repent of your sins, ask Jesus to forgive you of your sins, cleanse you with His blood, and save you. Then confess Jesus Christ as your Lord and Savior (Rom. 10:9–13).

Once you know Jesus, you receive the gift of the Holy Spirit who will guide you in your pathway of healing and reveal your Bible cure (Acts 2:38).

Before you close these pages of *The Bible Cure,* I want you to know that I am praying for you to serve the Lord all the days of your life, to stand firm, and finish strong your course with joy.

*Lord Jesus,*

*I pray for this precious reader right now, that Your Holy Spirit will guide him or her in a specific pathway of healing. By Your Spirit, give my friend the determination to apply the principles of* The Bible Cure *to his or her life so he or she will be able to worship and serve You with a healthy body, soul, and spirit— finishing the course with joy.*

*Amen.*

# Notes

## CHAPTER 1
### TRUTHS THAT AMAZED THIS SCIENTIST AND PHYSICIAN

1. Isadore Rosenfeld, M.D., *Dr. Rosenfeld's Guide to Alternative Medicine* (New York: Random House, 1996), 101.
2. Harris, Archer Jr., Waitke, eds., *Theological Wordbook of the Old Testament* (Chicago: Moody Bible Institute, 1980), 287.
3. Craig, Haigh, and Harrar, *The Complete Book of Alternative Nutrition,* edited by the editors of *Prevention Magazine* (Emmaus, PA: Rodale Press, Inc., 1997), 360.
4. *Taber Cyclopedic Medical Dictionary* (Philadelphia, PA: F. A. Davis Company, 1997), 841.
5. Jack Deere, *Surprised by the Power of the Spirit* (Grand Rapids, MI: Zondervan Publishing House, 1993), 57.
6. *Corpus Medicorum Graecorum* (vol. 4, 2, 246, 20), circa A.D. 130–200.

## CHAPTER 2
### GOD'S HEALING SECRETS IN THE OLD COVENANT

1. T. A. Burkill, "Medicine in Ancient Israel," *The Central African Journal of Medicine,* (July 1977), 153.
2. *Theological Wordbook,* 405.
3. George Cansdale, "Clean and Unclean Animals," *Eerdmans' Handbook to the Bible,* David and Pat Alexander, eds. (Grand Rapids, MI: William B. Eerdmans Publishing Company, 1973), 176.
4. Shaul G. Massry, Miroslaw Smogorzewski, Elizur Hazani, Shaul M. Shasha, "Influence of Judaism and Jewish Physicians

on Greek and Byzantine Medicine and Their Contribution to Nephrology," *American Journal of Nephrology*, vol. 17, Issue 3-4, (1997), 233.
5. L. M. Friedman, *Washington and Mosaic Law,* (American Jewish Historical Society, 1950), 24:320.
6. Summarized from the *Theological Dictionary of the New Testament,* Geoffrey W. Bromiley, ed. (Grand Rapids, MI: William B. Eerdmans Publishing Company, 1985), 1132ff.
7. Leonard F. Peltier, M.D., Ph.D., "Patron Saints of Medicine," *Clinical Orthopaedics and Related Research*, no. 334, 375.
8. Summarized from the *Theological Dictionary of the New Testament,* Geoffrey W. Bromiley, ed. (Grand Rapids, MI: William B. Eerdmans Publishing Company, 1985), 1202.
9. See *A Greek English Lexicon of the New Testament and Other Early Christian Literature,* W. F. Arndt and F. W. Gingrich, eds. (Chicago: University of Chicago Press, 1957), 368.

CHAPTER 5
HEALTHY EATING WITH THE MEDITERRANEAN DIET

1. *Everyday Life in Bible Times,* James B. Pritchard, ed. (National Geographic Society, 1967), 242, 332.
2. James I. Cook, *The Oxford Companion to the Bible,* Bruce M. Metzger, Michael D. Coogan, eds. (New York: Oxford University Press, 1993), s.v. "bread," 95.

# Appendix

# The Bible Cure's Healthy Recipes

L INDA AND I have been following the Mediterranean Diet eating plan for several years. Linda has developed many creative, tasty recipes, and we want to share some of our favorites with you.

⚜

## DR. CHERRY'S BREAKFAST CEREAL MIXTURE

⚜

$^1/_2$ cup Fiber One cereal
$^1/_3$ cup oat bran

Combine both cereals in a bowl and add fat-free milk.

❦

## LINDA'S BREAKFAST DRINK

❦

1 package Carnation Instant Diet Breakfast mix
$1/3$ cup oat bran

Mix together with 10 ounces fat-free (or 1- or 2-percent low-fat) milk. Drink through a straw, stirring occasionally.

❦

## STRAWBERRY-BANANA MILKSHAKE

❦

2 cups buttermilk
1 pint fresh hulled strawberries
2 ripe bananas
honey to taste

Blend all ingredients in a blender, adding 6 to 8 ice cubes as you blend the mixture. Sweeten to taste with honey.

❦

## OAT BRAN MUFFINS

❦

2 cups oat bran cereal
$1/4$ cup brown sugar, firmly packed
2 tsp. baking powder
1 cup fat-free (or 1- or 2-percent low-fat) milk
3 egg whites, beaten slightly
$1/4$ cup honey
2 Tbsp. extra-virgin olive or canola oil

Combine all ingredients. Mix well and pour mixture into 12 muffin cups lined with paper baking liners. Fill muffin cups $3/4$ full. Bake at 425 degrees for 15 to 17 minutes.

❧

## COLE SLAW

❧

¹/₂ cup Weight Watcher's fat-free whipped salad dressing
  (or fat-free mayonnaise)
¹/₂ tsp. white vinegar
1 Tbsp. extra-virgin olive or canola oil
3 Tbsp. fat-free (or 1- to 2-percent low-fat) milk
2 tsp. prepared mustard
4 packets of NutraSweet (Equal)
1 shredded head of cabbage
2 shredded carrots

Combine all ingredients except the cabbage and carrots. Whip the dressing ingredients with a wire whisk. Pour over shredded cabbage and carrots. Toss until well coated. Serves 6.

❧

## CAESAR SALAD

❧

¹/₄ cup extra-virgin olive oil
1 tsp. lemon juice (fresh or concentrate)
3–4 shakes of red wine vinegar
2 cloves minced garlic
1 squirt anchovy paste
several sprinkles of freshly ground black pepper
¹/₃ cup grated low-fat Parmesan cheese
8 romaine lettuce leaves
tomato or cucumber chunks (optional)

Separate lettuce leaves; rinse in cold water; blot dry; wrap in clean dish towel; and refrigerate for approximately thirty minutes. When ready to serve, tear lettuce into bite-size pieces for salad. Mix all dressing ingredients. Just before serving, pour the dressing over the lettuce and toss well. You may add tomatoes or cucumbers if desired. Serves 4–6.

❦

## TABOULI SALAD

❦

1 cup bulgur wheat
2 cups boiling water
$^3/_4$ cup fresh minced parsley
$^3/_4$ cup chopped green onions
$^3/_4$ cup cooked navy or garbanzo beans
1 cup diced cucumber
2 chopped tomatoes
3 Tbsp. fresh minced mint (or 1 tsp. each dried basil and oregano)
5 Tbsp. extra-virgin olive oil
5 Tbsp. fresh lemon juice
$^1/_2$ tsp. freshly ground black pepper
2 cloves minced garlic
1 small head romaine lettuce

SALAD: In a glass or metal mixing bowl, pour the boiling water over the bulgur wheat. Cover the bowl and let it stand for 1 hour. Drain the excess water off the wheat. Add the parsley, onions, beans, cucumber, tomatoes, and mint. Set aside.

DRESSING: Combine the olive oil, lemon juice, pepper, and garlic to make the dressing. Stir the dressing into the salad. Chill for at least one hour. Serve on a bed of whole lettuce leaves. Leaves may be rolled around the salad for eating as a finger food. Serves 6–8.

## TOMATOES ITALIANO

2 large halved tomatoes
3 Tbsp. shredded fresh basil (or 1 Tbsp. dried)
1–2 cloves minced garlic
Cracked black pepper
2 tsp. extra-virgin olive oil
low-fat Parmesan cheese

In a small bowl, combine the basil, garlic, pepper, and olive oil. Spread equally on top of tomato halves. Sprinkle lightly with Parmesan cheese. Place in a round glass dish and microwave on high for 3½ minutes. This is good with almost anything.

## VINAIGRETTE DRESSING

2 Tbsp. red wine vinegar
½ tsp. Morton Lite Salt
½ tsp. dry mustard
6 Tbsp. extra-virgin olive (or canola) oil
½ tsp. freshly ground black pepper

Combine all ingredients. Whip dressing with a wire whisk until smooth. Pour over chilled lettuce, tomatoes, and other salad vegetables of your choice. Toss until well coated. Serve immediately.

꧁꧂

## GARLIC-LEMON DRESSING

꧁꧂

3 Tbsp. extra-virgin olive oil
1 Tbsp. fresh lemon juice
$1/2$ garlic clove
1 tsp. Morton Lite Salt
Freshly ground black pepper to taste

In a clean, dry salad bowl, crush the garlic and salt together with a spoon to make a smooth paste. Add the lemon juice and stir until the salt is dissolved. Add the olive oil and pepper. Mix the dressing well.

This dressing, used in the eastern Mediterranean, is used on green salads as well as over steamed vegetables. It makes $1/4$ cup.

꧁꧂

## LOW-FAT LIME DRESSING

꧁꧂

2 Tbsp. lime juice
grated rind from 1 lime
$1/4$ cup nonfat mayonnaise
$1/4$ cup nonfat sour cream
2 Tbsp. honey
2 cups torn lettuce
2 Tbsp. chopped pecans, almonds, or walnuts

In a cup, whisk together the mayonnaise, sour cream, honey, grated rind from one lime, and the lime juice.

This is a low-fat, sweet-tart dressing. Serve with seasonal fruit variations. Suggested fruits to use in your own combinations are:

2 cups halved fresh figs
1 cup watermelon balls
1 cup blueberries
1 cup orange sections

1 cup sliced banana
1 cup cantaloupe balls
1 cup diced apple

Other fruits could include raspberries, strawberries, peaches, pears, or pineapples.

In a large bowl, toss your chosen fruit combination with one tablespoon lime juice. Let the fruit stand about five minutes to blend the flavors. Place the lettuce on individual plates and top with the fruit and dollops of dressing. Sprinkle with pecans, almonds, or walnuts.

## COOKING DRIED BEANS

Rinse 1 pound dried beans in a colander and discard any "bad" beans. Place remaining beans in a pot of cold water. Add 1 tablespoon Morton Lite Salt. Bring beans to a boil, then cover the pot and turn off the heat. Let set overnight. The next morning, cook the beans until they are tender (several hours), following the directions on the bean package.

There are many ingredients that can be added to beans, including turkey bones that you have saved (keep them frozen until using). Other ingredients include garlic, onions, celery, tomatoes, and cilantro. Herbs and spices that can be added include basil, ground pepper, cumin, oregano, thyme, rosemary, creole seasoning, and other favorites. This is one healthy way to cook beans. Dried bean varieties to use: great northern, navy, pinto, lima, black, and butter beans.

❧

## Pinto Beans Deluxe

❧

4–6 cups cooked pinto beans
1 medium chopped onion
1 16-oz. can stewed tomatoes
1 Tbsp. Mexican-style chili powder
1 handful fresh cilantro

Follow the directions on the dried bean package to cook the beans; just before the beans have finished cooking add the onion, tomatoes, chili powder, and handful of fresh cilantro.

❧

## My Favorite Greens

❧

3 Tbsp. extra-virgin olive oil, divided
1 large chopped onion
2 diced celery stalks
chopped greens (collard, turnip, mustard, spinach, or cabbage)
1 cup water
salt-free Mrs. Dash or Parsley Patch

Pour 2 tablespoons extra-virgin olive oil in the bottom of a stainless steel pot. Sauté onion and celery stalks in oil until tender. Place chopped collard, turnip, mustard greens, fresh spinach, or cabbage in pot. Add the water. Sprinkle the top of the greens with Mrs. Dash or Parsley Patch. Pour 1 tablespoon olive oil on top of the greens. Let cook about 5 minutes. Toss well. Cook on low heat, tossing occasionally until tender.

❧

## MEDITERRANEAN-STYLE BEAN SOUP

❧

2 Tbsp. extra-virgin olive oil
1 large chopped onion
3 medium peeled and chopped carrots
2 crushed garlic cloves
2 cups dried beans, soaked and drained
8 cups boiling water
1 14-oz. can stewed tomatoes with juice
1 Tbsp. fresh crumbled thyme (or 1 tsp. dried)
2 bay leaves
Approximately ¼ cup chopped parsley, plus some for garnish
Morton Lite Salt to taste
freshly ground black pepper to taste
Croutons for garnish (optional)

Soak the beans overnight, or prepare according to package directions. In a heavy three-quart stock pot, heat the olive oil and sauté the onion, carrots, and garlic until the vegetables are soft but not browned (about 10 minutes).

Add the drained beans and boiling water to soup pot; add thyme, bay leaves, and parsley. Cover and cook over low heat 1 to 3 hours, adding water occasionally as needed or until beans are soft (cooking time varies with type of beans).

When beans are soft, add the lite salt and pepper. For thicker soup, remove about 1½ cups of beans and purée in a food processor or blender. Return to pot. For thinner soup, add hot water. Garnish with chopped parsley or croutons. Experiment by using different kinds of beans each time you prepare this recipe.

❧

## Linda's Vegetable Soup

❧

1½ onions
1 green bell pepper
½ head of cabbage
3 celery stalks with leaves
4 carrots

Cut the vegetables into medium chunks. Add:

1 32-oz. can stewed tomatoes
1 tsp. minced garlic
1 tsp. thyme
1 Tbsp. Morton Lite Salt
½ tsp. freshly ground black pepper
6–8 dashes hot pepper sauce

The following vegetables are optional and could be added to your stock pot before cooking: yellow squash, zucchini squash, fresh Brussels sprouts, cauliflower florets.

Combine all ingredients in a large stock pot and bring to a boil. Reduce heat to medium and cook approximately 20 minutes or until the vegetables are tender.

❧

## Spaghetti Squash

❧

Cut spaghetti squash lengthwise and remove seeds.

CONVENTIONAL OVEN METHOD: Bake squash, cut side down, in shallow baking dish sprayed with olive oil or canola no-stick cooking spray at 350 degrees for 45 minutes.

MICROWAVE OVEN METHOD: Bake squash, cut side down, in shallow baking dish with ¼ cup water. Cover with clear plastic wrap. Make several slits in wrap. Cook on high for 7 to 10 minutes.

Remove from oven. Use a fork to scrape the inside of the squash, creating spaghetti-like strands of cooked squash. Add Morton Lite Salt, freshly ground black pepper, and fat-free margarine, if desired.

## EASTERN YELLOW SQUASH CASSEROLE

$^1/_2$ cup nonfat yogurt
$^1/_2$ cup nonfat cottage cheese
$^1/_2$ cup fat-free egg substitute (or 2 eggs)
$^1/_4$ cup grated low-fat Parmesan cheese
$^1/_4$ tsp. dried marjoram
1 cup thinly sliced onions
3 cups thinly sliced yellow squash
$^1/_4$ cup fresh whole wheat bread crumbs

In a small bowl, blend the yogurt, cottage cheese, eggs (yes, eggs), Parmesan cheese, and marjoram. Set aside.

Coat a large nonstick frying pan with a no-cholesterol, no-stick cooking spray. Add the onions and cook over medium heat for 5 minutes. Coat a 2-quart casserole dish with the same no-stick spray. Spread $^1/_3$ of the squash slices in the dish. Top with $^1/_3$ of the onions and $^1/_3$ of the yogurt mixture. Repeat the layers twice. Sprinkle top with the bread crumbs.

Cover with aluminum foil and bake at 375 degrees for 20 minutes. Uncover and bake for 5 minutes, or until the bread crumbs are golden brown. This simple casserole is excellent with baked fish or baked chicken.

❦

## BAKED OR BROILED FISH

❦

BAKED FISH: Fresh fish generally takes about 20 minutes to bake. If the fish is cut thick, it may take a little longer. Place fish in a baking dish that has been sprayed with olive oil or canola oil no-stick cooking spray to avoid sticking. It is not necessary to turn the fish over while baking.

BROILED FISH: Fresh fish generally takes about 5 to 7 minutes per side to broil. Appearance is the indicator. Place fish in a microwave dish that has been sprayed with olive oil or canola oil no-stick cooking spray to avoid sticking.

HEALTHY TOPPINGS FOR BAKED OR BROILED FISH: Mrs. Dash or Parsley Patch (salt-free), lemon, Fines herbs, Italian herb seasoning, crushed oregano leaves, freshly ground black pepper, crushed parsley leaves, and creole seasonings (salt-free).

❦

## BROILED SALMON STEAKS

❦

1 salmon steak per person
Fines herbs or Italian herb seasoning
olive oil

Place the salmon steaks on a broiler pan or cookie sheet covered with aluminum foil or in a shallow baking dish sprayed with olive oil or canola no-stick cooking spray. Sprinkle the tops of the steaks with Fines herbs or Italian herb seasoning. Put a few drops of olive oil in the center of each steak. Broil on the first side for 5 to 7 minutes. Turn the steaks over, sprinkle with seasoning, dot with olive oil, and broil on the second side for 5 to 7 minutes. Serve immediately.

Serving suggestion: Broiled salmon is good with rice or baked potato, broccoli, and salad.

❧

# ALASKAN SALMON 'N' RICE

❧

2 cups cooked brown rice
1 can (7³/₄ oz.) drained salmon, reserving liquid
1 cup chopped onion
¹/₂ cup chopped celery
¹/₂ cup chopped bell pepper
3 Tbsp. extra-virgin olive oil
¹/₂–1 tsp. curry powder
1 10-oz. package frozen chopped broccoli, thawed and
    drained, or 10-oz. fresh
dash of freshly ground black pepper

Cook the brown rice according to package directions. Set aside. Drain and flake the salmon, reserving the liquid. Add enough water to the reserved liquid to total ¹/₃ cup. Sauté onion, celery, green pepper, and curry powder in the olive oil. Add salmon, rice, broccoli, and reserved salmon liquid. Mix well. Season with dash of pepper. Spray baking dish with olive oil or canola no-stick cooking spray; spread ingredients in the dish. Cover with aluminum foil and bake at 350 degrees for 25 to 30 minutes. Serves 4 to 6 persons.

꧁❦꧂

## ITALIAN SALMON AND PASTA DINNER

꧁❦꧂

8 ounces fettuccine noodles, or pasta of choice
1 cup sliced mushrooms
1 cup sliced onions
1 Tbsp. extra-virgin olive oil
1 cup diced tomatoes
1 can (12–14 oz.) salmon, drained and flaked
$\frac{1}{4}$ cup nonfat chicken broth
pinch of hot pepper flakes
2 Tbsp. fresh minced basil
3 Tbsp. grated low-fat Parmesan cheese

In a large no-stick frying pan, sauté the mushrooms and onions in the olive oil over medium-high heat for 5 minutes. Add the tomatoes, salmon, broth, and pepper flakes. Cover and simmer over low heat for 5 minutes.

While you are cooking the salmon ingredients prepare the pasta. Cook the fettuccine noodles in a large pot of boiling water for 10 minutes or until tender. Drain and place on individual plates or a large platter. Add the salmon mixture and basil; toss well to combine. Sprinkle with the Parmesan cheese.

This is a simple dish to prepare. Serve with a dinner salad or a Caesar salad and fruit for a complete meal.

꧁꧂

# MEDITERRANEAN SPINACH ENCHILADAS

꧁꧂

1$\frac{1}{2}$ cups nonfat chicken broth
1 cup diced mild canned green chili peppers
2 diced tomatoes
2 Tbsp. finely chopped onions
2 cloves minced garlic
2 Tbsp. cornstarch
2 Tbsp. water
1$\frac{1}{4}$ lb. fresh chopped spinach
8 corn tortillas

In a 2-quart saucepan, combine the broth, chili peppers, tomatoes, onions, and garlic. Bring to a boil. Simmer over low heat for 15 minutes.

In a small bowl, combine the cornstarch and water. Add to the broth and continue cooking, stirring as the mixture cooks until it thickens. Remove from the heat.

While the sauce is cooking, steam the spinach for 5 minutes. Coat a 9- by 13-inch baking dish with a no-cholesterol, no-stick cooking spray. Divide the spinach equally among the tortillas and roll, placing a single layer of enchiladas in the baking dish with the open side down. Top with the tomato mixture. Bake at 400 degrees for 10 minutes. This tasty dish will make a complete meal when served with a salad.

❦

## CHICKEN AND GREEN RICE

❦

1 whole chicken
2-14$^1/_2$ oz. cans nonfat chicken broth
2 cups brown rice
3 Tbsp. extra-virgin olive oil
2 stalks diced celery
1 medium diced onion
1 diced green bell pepper
2 Tbsp. parsley flakes
1 tsp. Morton Lite Salt
$^1/_2$ tsp. freshly ground black pepper

Boil one whole chicken and remove the bones. Following the rice package directions, cook the rice in the broth, adding enough water to make 4 cups of liquid.

Pour the olive oil in a skillet. Sauté the bell pepper, celery, and onion until tender. Add the parsley flakes, lite salt, and pepper. Combine this mixture with the cooked rice. Add the chicken and mix well. (For variation add 1 to 2 teaspoons poultry seasoning and mix well.) Spray a 9- by 13-inch baking dish with olive oil or canola oil no-stick cooking spray. Spread ingredients in the dish. Cover with aluminum foil. Bake at 350 degrees for 45 minutes. Serves 6 to 8 persons.

❧

## BAKED CHICKEN IN A BAG

❧

1 whole chicken
$\frac{1}{2}$ cup each of diced celery, onion, and carrots
low-calorie Italian dressing

Stuff a whole chicken with fresh celery, onion, and carrot pieces. Coat the outside skin with low-calorie Italian salad dressing. Place the chicken in a browning bag and place in a 9- by 13-inch baking dish. Make six half-inch slits in the top of the bag. Bake at 350 degrees for 45 to 50 minutes. Remove the skin before eating.

❧

## UNCLE CHARLES' SKILLET CHICKEN

❧

2 uncooked packaged chicken breast fillets
1 medium chopped onion
freshly ground black pepper
1 Tbsp. extra-virgin olive oil

Pour 1 tablespoon olive oil in a skillet. Add 1 medium chopped onion. Cut the chicken fillets into cubes and add to the skillet. Sprinkle with freshly ground black pepper. Stir and cook until chicken is white and tender, about 10 minutes. Serve immediately over rice, pasta, or potatoes. Serves 4.

꙳

## Healthiest Fried Chicken

꙳

1 whole chicken, skinned and cut up
1-1½ cups whole-wheat flour
¼ tsp. Morton Lite Salt
¼ tsp. freshly ground black pepper
canola oil

Heat enough oil in a skillet to fry the chicken. Combine flour, salt, and pepper in a 1-gallon plastic bag. Shake to mix ingredients. Rinse chicken with water. Place chicken pieces in plastic bag and shake well to coat chicken on all sides. Cook in hot oil until golden brown, turning as needed.

Serving suggestion: This chicken is good with corn on the cob, mashed potatoes, steamed vegetables, salad, and especially good with cole slaw. This is a southern delight!

Cooking note: Whole-wheat flour browns more quickly than white flour. Fry chicken on medium-high heat, turning as needed. Watch carefully to ensure that chicken is done.